THE INTERPROFESSIONAL HEALTH CARE TEAM

LEADERSHIP AND DEVELOPMENT

THIRD EDITION

Donna Weiss, PhD, FAOTA

Emeritus Faculty
Occupational Therapy Program
Department of Health and Rehabilitation Sciences
College of Public Health
Temple University
Philadelphia, PA

Felice J. Tilin, PhD, PCC

Associate Adjunct Professor, University of Pennsylvania
President, GroupWorks Consulting LLC

Marlene J. Morgan, Ed.D, OTR/L

Associate Professor
Department of Occupational Therapy
The University of Scranton, Scranton, PA

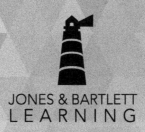

JONES & BARTLETT
LEARNING

World Headquarters
Jones & Bartlett Learning
25 Mall Road
Burlington, MA 01803
978-443-5000
info@jblearning.com
www.jblearning.com

Jones & Bartlett Learning books and products are available through most bookstores and online booksellers. To contact Jones & Bartlett Learning directly, call 800-832-0034, fax 978-443-8000, or visit our website, www.jblearning.com.

27341-0

Production Credits
Vice President, Product Management: Marisa R. Urbano
Vice President, Content Strategy and Implementation:
   Christine Emerton
Director, Product Management: Matthew Kane
Product Manager: Bill Lawrensen
Director, Content Management: Donna Gridley
Content Strategist: Ashley Malone
Director, Project Management and Content Services:
   Karen Scott
Manager, Project Management: Jackie Reynen
Project Manager: Erin Bosco
Program Manager: Alex Schab
Senior Digital Project Specialist: Carolyn Downer
Marketing Manager: Mark Adamiak
Content Services Manager: Colleen Lamy
Product Fulfillment Manager: Wendy Kilborn
Composition: Straive
Project Management: Straive
Cover and Text Design: Kristin E. Parker
Media Development Editor: Faith Brosnan
Rights & Permissions Manager: John Rusk
Rights Specialist: Robin Landry
Cover Image (Title Page, Part Opener, Chapter Opener):
   © oxygen/Moment/Getty Images
Printing and Binding: Gasch Printing

Library of Congress Cataloging-in-Publication Data
Names: Weiss, Donna (Donna F.), author. | Tilin, Felice J., author. |
   Morgan, Marlene J., author.
Title: The interprofessional health care team : leadership and development
   / Donna Weiss, Felice Tilin, Marlene Morgan.
Description: Third edition. | Burlington, Massachusetts : Jones & Bartlett
   Learning, [2024] | Includes bibliographical references and index. |
   Identifiers: LCCN 2023012339 | ISBN 9781284273380 (paperback)
Subjects: MESH: Patient Care Team–organization & administration |
   Leadership
Classification: LCC RA971 | NLM W 84.8 | DDC 610.68–dc23/eng/20230620
LC record available at https://lccn.loc.gov/2023012339

6048

Printed in the United States of America
26 25 24 23 22 10 9 8 7 6 5 4 3 2 1

Brief Contents

Contents

PART I Team and Group Development ... 1

Preface

Anthony J. Mazzarelli, MD, JD, MBE
Co-CEO Cooper University Health Care
Coauthor of *Compassionomics:*
The Revolutionary Scientific Evidence
That Caring Makes a Difference

Kevin M. O'Dowd, JD
Co-CEO Cooper University Health Care
Former U.S. Department of Justice
Federal Health Care Fraud Prosecutor
Former Counsel and Chief of Staff to the
Governor, State of New Jersey

As you begin your journey through this book about interprofessional healthcare teams, you will be introduced to a wealth of information and insights about the nature of collaboration, cooperation, and the role of leadership across the many different fields of expertise in health care. You will learn about the unique challenges and opportunities that arise when individuals with diverse professional and social backgrounds come together to tackle complex problems, as well as strategies and best practices for fostering successful interprofessional teams.

As co-CEOs of Cooper University Health Care, we are an interprofessional team between ourselves as well as with our executive leadership. We have very different backgrounds between the two of us. We recognized early in our tenure that we need to be aligned as a team and that we need to support teams from executives through care teams to work across professions to provide optimal patient care.

Whether you are a team leader looking to assemble a group of experts from different disciplines, or a member of an interprofessional team seeking to improve patient care, this book will provide you with valuable insights and practical advice. With the growing importance of interprofessional collaboration in today's rapidly changing world, this book is a must-read for anyone seeking to understand and harness the power of diverse perspectives and expertise.

This book will continue to be an important resource with stimulating questions that will inspire both novices and experts to think differently about their roles and styles as leaders or members of a team. This third edition has expanded sections on diversity and inclusion, relational leadership, and facilitating collaborative cultures with examples of how to create compassionate dialogue and psychological safety in virtual settings. The authors provide many tools to empower readers and facilitate the fostering of productive teamwork. It is an inspiring book with easily operational principles. Our gratitude goes out to the authors for having the wisdom, knowledge, and experience to invest in writing and updating this book. It is written for many audiences and to achieve many goals all centered on best practices to attain quality care, particularly during this time of reinventing and transforming health care.

Acknowledgments

Our individual contributions to this book are products of the innumerable relationships that we have been fortunate enough to enjoy over the course of our professional and personal lives. Through our collaboration on this book, we have been edified and transformed by the experiences of each other. We share the deepest gratitude for the thought, guidance, and support that we have received from the following people:

To mentors: Annie McKee, Susan A. Wheelan, and Sherene Zolno, who generously shared their scholarship and fostered our learning.

To colleagues, teachers, clients, friends, and family for sharing their stories and wisdom: Rebecca Austill-Clausen, Stephen Berg, Marco Bertola, Joanne Broder Summerson, Tracy Christopherson, Luis Constantino, Claire Conway, Wanda Cooper, Laurie Cousart, Vincent Curren, Dan Drake, Mario DiCioccio, Peter Doukas, Tim Fox, Kevin Hook, Francis Johnston, Emily Keshner, Moya Kinnealey, John Kirby, Robin Kurilko, Delores Mason, Afaf Meleis, Karen Nichols, Linda Paolini, Prem Rawat, Debra Pellegrino, Melanie Rothschild, Carol L. Savrin, Stephen Scardina, Lana Schuette, Kathryn Shaffer, Judith Shamian, Carole Simon, Mary Sinnott, Beth Sippola, Rob Sippola, Trudi Sippola, David M. Smith, Eileen Sullivan-Marx, Bruce Theriault, Kelsey Tilin, Sam Tilin, Beulah Trey, and Sue Carol Verrillo.

To the team at Jones & Bartlett Learning who patiently provided support, advice, and encouragement throughout the publication process: William Lawrensen, Ashley Malone, Robin Silverman, Faith Brosnan, Erin Bosco, Mark Adamiak, and Padmapriya Soundararajan, Kevinesh Neeraj, and Sheryl Nelson. Special thanks are extended to Felice's colleagues at St. Joseph's University who provided the time and encouragement to complete this book: Karin Botto, Jeanne Brady, Sabrina DeTurk, William Madges, Robert Palestini, Becky Rice, Erin Schwing, and Wendy Thruman.

Finally, we acknowledge all learners—whether they are students, teachers, leaders, or group members—and their active engagement in asking questions and trying on new ways of thinking, being, and doing.

About the Authors

Donna Weiss, PhD, FAOTA, is a coach, trainer, and facilitator in the areas of interpersonal communication, group dynamics, and leadership in health care.

Felice J. Tilin, PhD, is an organization development consultant, facilitator, executive coach, and educator with multinational, private and nonprofit businesses, and healthcare organizations in the United States, Canada, Europe, Africa, and Asia.

Marlene J. Morgan, EdD, OTR/L, has extensive experience in clinical and academic leadership positions and her research interests include interprofessional education for health professionals.

Reviewers

Kim Amer, PhD, RN
DePaul University

Barbara Jean Braband, RN, EdD, CNE
University of Portland

Randy L. Byington, EdD, MBA
East Tennessee State University

Wanda Cloet, DHSC, RDH
Central Community College

Eileen Coughlin, MPA, MBA, SPHR
California State University—East Bay

Arleen Crutcher, PhD, MSN, RN
Colorado Christian University

Ann Curtis, DNP, RN
Maine College of Health Professions

Christina Daley, PhD, NHA
Pennsylvania State University

Tara Davis, PhD
University of South Alabama

Sherry DelGrosso, DNP, RN, LNC
St. Francis University

Regina Enwefa, PhD, ND
Southern University and A&M College

Harold Felton, DHEd/PA-C
Touro College

Kim Garcia, MED, RRT-NPS
University of Texas Rio Grande Valley

William Gordon, DMin, MDiv
Rosalind Franklin University of Medicine
   and Science

Dana Griffin, MBA, MLS(ASCP)cm
Madonna University

Robert Hawkes, MSPA, PA-C
Florida Gulf Coast University

Matthew Kutz, PhD, ATC
Florida International University

Mackenzie Lanham, MSN, BS, RN, CLC
University of Charleston

Wei-Chen Lee, PhD
University of Texas Medical Branch

Jennifer Malone, OTD, MS, OTR/L
Moravian University

Samantha Marocco, PT, DPT, MS
Utica College

Jeffery V. McMinn, RDH, MA
Hudson Valley Community College

Michelle Morgan, MS, RDN, CDN
Russell Sage College

Jayme L. Ober, OTD, OTR.L, MSCS
Alvernia University

Tony Palmer, DBA
UNTHSC System College of Pharmacy

Travis Pollen, PhD
Jefferson University

Yasser Salem, PT, PhD, NCS, PCS
Hofstra University

Brandy Schneider, EdD, ATC
Truman State University

Shannon Schoellig, OTD, MS, OTR/L
Utica College

Teresa Seefeldt, PharmaD, PhD
South Dakota State University College of
   Pharmacy and Allied Health Professions

Melissa M. Snyder, PhD, LAT, ATC, CSCS
Western Carolina University

Angela Reed Summer, MPA, MSN, RN, CVRN-BC
Carlow University

Melissa K. Travelsted, DNP, APRN
Western Kentucky University

Peggy Ann Ursuy, PhD, MA, RN, PPCNP-BC
University of Michigan, School of Nursing

Kelli Whitted, DNP, FNP-BC
Troy University

Introduction: Interprofessional Leadership in the Healthcare Environment

LEARNING OBJECTIVES

1. Understand the interprofessional healthcare team as a broadly inclusionary concept.
2. Describe how an interprofessional orientation can enhance patient care.
3. Explain the importance of relationship-centered care to patient outcomes.
4. Understand the concept of members as leaders.

Human beings are social by nature and bond together in families, small groups, and tribes. As we attempt to navigate from childhood through adulthood, our behaviors tend to mirror those of our family groups, peer groups, and professional groups. As we mature, our sense of self is created in part by our interactions with and feedback from these groups. Over the millennia, interaction with a variety of other people has been necessary to fulfill primary needs like love and affection but also to accomplish the work inherent to community building and survival. With the evolution of societies from the Stone Age through the Information Age, the complexity of the challenges that individuals and organizations face has increased, as well as the need for well-functioning, diverse groups that can meet those challenges. Solving complex problems requires diverse information sets that are not the purview of a single person or a

single profession. This is true in all modern endeavors but most apparent in the healthcare industry.

The concept of health incorporates a complex and holistic system where biological, psychological, physical, socioeconomic, cultural, and environmental factors function as interconnected and interacting determinants of one another. Rowe (2003) has noted that health issues are characteristically broad and complex and are most appropriately examined from an interdisciplinary perspective. Reports from the Pew Health Professions Commission (1998), the Institute of Medicine (2001, 2002, 2003, 2015), and the World Health Organization (2010) have repeatedly supported the notion that educational programs for health professionals can only be considered complete if they include experiences working in interprofessional teams. The literature regarding higher education is replete with references to interdisciplinary, interprofessional, and integrative studies (Interprofessional Education Collaborative, 2016). External funding sources for research identify evidence of interprofessional collaboration as a key criterion for grant eligibility (Bray et al., 2007; García & Roblin, 2008; Palincsar, 2007). Evidence of interprofessional team experiences is included in the accreditation standards for many health professional education programs with the expectation that health professionals will be educated with an interprofessional orientation and will develop an ability to leverage the power of teams to solve complex problems (Frenk et al., 2010; Interprofessional Education Collaborative, 2016; Royeen et al., 2009).

Members of interprofessional healthcare teams work within increasingly complex organizational and political structures with multiple reporting relationships and competing value systems. The competitive healthcare market presents professionals with a variety of leadership challenges—not the least of which is learning to leverage the power of interdisciplinarity. Drinka and Clark (2000) define an interdisciplinary health care team (IHCT) as "a group of individuals with diverse training and backgrounds who work together as an identified unit or system" (p. 6). Disciplinary expertise is maximized when members of the IHCT can routinely employ strong relational skills and effectively coordinate their work with others. Relational coordination in the form of high-quality communication, mutual positive regard, trust, and active engagement are associated with a stronger collective identity, reduction in status differential, increased ability to respond to pressures with resilience, job satisfaction, and retention of staff. Most importantly, organizations that institutionalize the consistent communication strategies associated with relationship-centered organizations are high performing and profitable, have low employee turnover, better clinical outcomes, a reduction in length of stay, and enhanced

patient-perceived quality care (Gittell, 2009; Suchman et al., 2011; Uhlig & Raboin, 2015; Edmondson, 2019).

The trend toward specialization in the health professions may lead to a less inclusionary interpretation of Drinka and Clark's definition of interdisciplinarity. It may be interpreted as the inclusion of persons who have the same basic training but have a specialty. For instance, some people may consider an internist, gynecologist, and a physiatrist to be an interdisciplinary team. The term *interprofessional* connotes a broader perspective and may include persons who have professional licensure or certification in nursing, occupational therapy, physical therapy, speech and language pathology, social work, and other health-related professions in addition to physicians (Hammick et al., 2009). In literature and in practice, the terms are often used interchangeably.

Health care evolved from a hierarchical process dominated by physicians to an inclusionary team of professionals that was broadened to include patients and caregivers. The conceptual shift regarding the focus of health care occurred in tandem with the recognition of health care as a complex system of relationships. Neither term—*interdisciplinary* nor *interprofessional*—reflects the importance of the patient and other important constituencies/contexts in the achievement of positive patient outcomes. The more cogent term seems to be *relationship-centered*. The notion of relationship-centered healthcare teams reaches beyond the traditional core of physicians, nurses, and therapists and incorporates all the constituencies who impact patient outcomes. It implies that the construction of healthcare teams is unique to the individual patient needs. The breakdown of traditional professional boundaries is necessary to meet the challenge of providing widely accessible, quality and cost-effective health care (Grant et al., 1995; Nundy, 2021). Skills in team building, team membership, and the understanding of the group dynamics are foundational and indispensable for the next generation of healthcare leaders (Burtscher et al., 2020; Schot et al., 2020).

Whether teams are called interdisciplinary, interprofessional, or relationship centered, each member of the healthcare team needs to ask these important questions:

- Who needs to be involved in order for the best patient outcomes to be achieved?
- How can we work together to achieve those outcomes efficiently and effectively?
- What is my unique professional and personal contribution to the team?
- How can I facilitate the optimum functioning of the team and the best client outcomes?

The full potential of the interprofessional healthcare team is realized when each member assumes a leadership stance, recognizes the power of unique professional expertise and personal qualities, and actively contributes to relationship-centered, safe, effective, and quality health services. The designated leader is responsible for drawing out the leadership stance in all team members by modeling self-awareness, self-regulation, empathy, and positive communication and encouraging these behaviors in others (Boyatzis & McKee, 2005). Leaders who are successful in facilitating a proactive leadership stance throughout their teams realize that their own perspective is incomplete and recognize the value of engaging the wisdom and power of the collective. In doing so, they create sustainable, relationship-centered, and highly productive team cultures that are creatively resilient in the face of change and thrive over time (Uhlig & Raboin, 2015; Hu et al., 2016).

Leadership in the interprofessional healthcare team means that both the designated leader and members must be willing to share the responsibilities of team leadership and be cognizant of group dynamics in order to work with widely diverse skills, values, and interests

(Lee, 2010). Appropriately addressing these issues requires strong leadership that has a broad and integrative perspective. Leadership should be embraced by a cadre of professionals who leverage their own disciplinary knowledge base and integrate it with those of other related disciplines in order to develop advanced understanding and competence in patient-centered and relationship-centered practice (Burtscher et al., 2020; Schot et al., 2020). The accountability for this type of leadership is shared by health professionals, at all organizational levels, who engage in research, teaching, health administration, and health policy development, as well as direct patient care (Boucher, 2016).

The challenge facing health professionals is that while most health professionals work in interprofessional teams and recognize their value, the majority have been professionally acculturated into their respective professional guilds rather than seeing themselves as members of a team. Until recently, professional training in most of the health disciplines did not emphasize collaboration, group decision-making, or shared leadership (Calhoun et al., 2008; Lee, 2010). The Institute of Medicine reported that a lack of effective collaboration among disciplines was most often identified as the cause of medical errors (Institute of Medicine, 1999, 2003). For example, a boy dies of a treatable infection or pain-reducing palliative care is withheld from a terminally ill patient for want of communication between doctors and other care givers (Dowd, 2012; Brown, 2012). On the other hand, effective interprofessional collaboration is linked to improved patient outcomes (Wheelan et al., 2003; Hu et al., 2016; Schot et al., 2020; Burtscher et al., 2020). "It is becoming increasingly apparent the effort to produce high quality care is not hampered by lack of clinical expertise in the individual professions but rather by lack of appropriate knowledge and experience among these groups as to how to make these multidisciplinary teams work well" (Freshman, Rubino, & Chassiakos, 2010, p. 6).

As health systems increase in complexity, health professionals need to develop confidence in group problem-solving, successful conflict management and resolution, efficient and effective information exchange, and boundary management (Gray, 2008; McKinlay et al., 2015). These competencies dependent on an understanding of the stages of group development and what makes teams effective. An effective team shows high levels of reflectivity and self-management skill, the ability to develop and maintain reciprocal relationships, and the willingness to empower others (Goleman & Boyatzis, 2008). The most successful and productive healthcare teams are those in which the concept of the collective as leader is applied. This means that all members, regardless of status, are self-aware and committed to assuming leadership and responsibility for the continued development of the group (Institute of Medicine, 2015).

While this book is designed primarily as a textbook, it is also useful as a guide for clinical team management. Additionally, individual health professionals may use the experiential activities and reflections to facilitate their own personal leadership capacity. The authors hope that readers will use this book to foster knowledge, skills, and attitudes that will enable them to be positive agents of change and growth in themselves, others, and their organizations. This text is composed of three parts: Teamwork and Group Development, Relationship-Centered Leadership, and Building and Sustaining Collaborative Interprofessional Teams. Each part is divided into chapters that introduce theoretical concepts and provide case stories and active teaching/learning experiences that are appropriate for in-class, online, or personal reflective learning environments. Teaching and learning activities are informed primarily by Kolb's model of adult learning and are designed to encourage reflection, dialogue, and the application of new knowledge into everyday practice (Kolb, 2015).

Part I: Teamwork and Group Development draws on classic group dynamic research to introduce groups as complex systems and relates foundational group dynamics concepts to interprofessional healthcare groups and teams. This section includes models of group dynamics, the developmental stages of groups, and how to optimize teamwork throughout the group life-span. Activities provide practice in differentiating personal from group goals, analyzing the developmental levels of groups, and applying strategies that individual leaders/members can employ to foster and sustain highly functional teams.

Part II: Relationship-Centered Leadership provides a detailed discussion of leadership behaviors, emotional intelligence, and how self-awareness, self-management, and an understanding of positive psychology can facilitate team development and productivity. Activities will help the reader analyze competencies required for health professions leadership; analyze leadership behaviors in real-life situations; identify personal leadership characteristics, challenges, philosophy, and behaviors; and conceptualize strategies for successful personal and health professional leadership for members as well as leaders of healthcare teams.

Part III: Building and Sustaining Collaborative Interprofessional Teams focuses on employing generative practices to appreciate diversity in all its forms, span professional boundaries, and facilitate the development of a team culture. Generative practices such as appreciative inquiry and positive communication can facilitate the development of affiliative environments and help sustain the productivity and effectiveness of relationship-centered healthcare teams. Real-world profiles provide examples of these concepts in action. Activities will focus on helping the reader develop interpersonal sensitivity, utilize empathic communication, give and receive feedback, use positive influence to build trust, manage conflict, and leverage the creativity and energy of diverse healthcare teams.

References

Boucher, N. A. (2016). Direct engagement with communities and interprofessional learning to factor culture into end-of-life health care delivery. *American Journal of Public Health.* doi: 10.2105/AJPH.2016.303073

Boyatzis, R., & McKee, A. (2005). *Resonant leadership.* Harvard Business School Press.

Bray, M., Adamson, B., & Mason, M. (Eds.). (2007). *Comparative education research: Approaches and methods.* Hong Kong China: Comparative Education Research Centre.

Brown, T. (2012, July 15). The boy who wanted to fly. *New York Times*, p. SR11.

Burtscher, M. J., Nussbeck, F. W., Sevdalis, N., Gisin, S., & Manser, T. (2020). Coordination and communication in healthcare action teams: The role of expertise. *Swiss Journal of Psychology, 79*(3-4), 123–135. https://doi.org/10.1024/1421-0185/a000239

Calhoun, J., Dollett, L., Sinioris, M., Wainio, J., Butler, P., Griffith, J., & Warden, G. (2008). Development of an interprofessional competency model for healthcare leadership. *Journal of Healthcare Management, 53*(6), 360–374.

Dowd, M. (2012, July 15). Don't get sick in July. *New York Times*, p. A20.

Drinka, T., & Clark, P. (2000). *Health care teamwork: Interdisciplinary practice and teaching.* Auburn House.

Edmondson, A. (2019). *The fearless organization.* Wiley.

Frenk, J., Chen, L., Bhutta, Z., Cohen, J., Crisp, N., & Zurayk, H. (2010). Health professionals for a new century: Transforming education to strengthen health systems in an interdependent world. *Lancet, 376*(9765), 1923–1958. doi:10.1016/S0140-6736(10)61854-5

Freshman, B., Rubino, L., & Chassiako, Y. (2010). *Collaboration across the disciplines in health care.* Jones & Bartlett Publishers.

García, L. M., & Roblin, N. P. (2008). Innovation, research and professional development in higher education: Learning from our own experience. *Teaching and Teacher Education, 24*(1), 104–116.

Gittell, J. (2009). *High performance healthcare: Using the power of relationships to achieve quality, efficiency and resilience.* McGraw Hill.

Goleman, D., & Boyatzis, R. (2008). Social intelligence and the biology of leadership. *Harvard Business Review, 86*(9), 74–81.

Grant, R. W., Finocchio, L. J., & California Primary Care Consortium Subcommittee on Interdisciplinary Collaboration. (1995). *Interdisciplinary collaborative teams in primary care: A model curriculum and resource guide.* Pew Health Professions Commission.

Gray, B. (2008). Enhancing transdisciplinary research through collaborative leadership. *American Journal of Preventive Medicine, 35*(2S), s124–s132.

Hammick, M., Freeth, D. S., Copperman, J., & Goodsman, D. (2009). *Being interprofessional.* Polity Press.

Hu, Y., Parker, S. H., Lipsitz, S. R., Arriaga, A. F., Peyre, S. E., Corso, K. A., Roth, E. M., Yule, S. J., & Greenberg, C. C. (2016). Surgeons' leadership styles and team behavior in the operating room. *Journal of the American College of Surgeons, 222*(1), 41–51. doi: 10.1016/j.jamcollsurg.2015.09.013

Institute of Medicine. (1999). *To err is human: Building a safer health system.* National Academies Press.

Institute of Medicine. (2001). *Crossing the quality chasm: A new health system for the 21st century.* National Academies Press.

Institute of Medicine. (2002). *Who will keep the public healthy? Educating public health professionals for the 21st century.* National Academies Press.

Institute of Medicine. (2003). *Health professions education: A bridge to quality.* National Academies Press.

Institute of Medicine. (2015). *Measuring the impact of interprofessional education on collaborative practice and patient outcomes.* National Academies Press.

Interprofessional Education Collaborative Expert Panel. (2011). *Core competencies for interprofessional collaborative practice: Report of an expert panel.* Author.

Interprofessional Education Collaborative. (2016). *Core competencies for interprofessional collaborative practice: 2016 update.* Author.

Kolb, D. (2015). *Experiential learning: Experience as the source of learning and development* (2nd ed.). Pearson Education.

Lee, T. (2010). Turning doctors into leaders. *Harvard Business Review, 88*(4), 50–58.

McKinlay, E., Gallagher, M. P., Gray, L., Wilson, C., & Pullon, S. (2015). Sixteen months "from square one": The process of forming an interprofessional clinical teaching team. *Journal of Research in Interprofessional Practice and Education, 5*(2). http://www.jripe.org/index.php/journal/article/view/191/119

Nundy, S. (2021). *Care after COVID: What the pandemic revealed is broken in health care and how to reinvent it.* McGraw Hill.

Palincsar, A. (2007). Reflections on the special issue. *Educational Psychology Review, 19*(1), 85–89.

Pew Health Professions Commission. (1998). *Recreating health professional practice for a new century: The fourth report of the Pew Health Professions Commission.* Author.

Rowe, J. (2003). Approaching interdisciplinary research. In F. Kessel, P. Rosenfield, & N. Anderson (Eds.), *Expanding the boundaries of health and social science: Case studies in interdisciplinary innovation* (pp. 3–9). Oxford University Press.

Royeen, C., Jensen, G., & Harvan, R. (2009). *Leadership in inter-disciplinary health care education and practice.* Jones & Bartlett Publishers.

Schot, E., Tummers, L., & Noordegraaf, M. (2020). Working on working together. A systematic review on how healthcare professionals contribute to interprofessional collaboration. *Journal of Interprofessional Care, 34*(3), 332–342. doi: 10.1080/13561820.2019.1636007

Suchman, A., Sluyter, D., & Williamson, P. (2011). *Leading change in healthcare: Transforming organizations using complexity, positive psychology and relationship-centered care.* London, England: Radcliffe Publishing.

Uhlig, P., & Raboin, W. E. (2015). *Field guide to collaborative care: Implementing the future of healthcare.* Oak Park Prairie Press.

Wheelan, S. A., Burchill, C. N., & Tilin, F. (2003). The link between teamwork and patients' outcomes in intensive care units. *American Journal of Critical Care, 12,* 527–534.

World Health Organization: Health Professions Network Nursing and Midwifery Office within the Department of Human Resources for Health. (2010). *Framework for action on interprofessional education & collaborative practice (WHO/HRH/HPN/10.3).* Geneva Switzerland: World Health Organization. http://www.who.int/hrh/nursing_midwifery/en/

© oxygen/Moment/Getty Images

Team and Group Development

"By recognizing our need to join with others…we have the opportunity for collective wisdom to emerge and facilitate the creation of new connections and innovative strategies to ensure the health and stability of the world that we share."

— Donna Weiss

CHAPTER 1

Groups-Teams-Systems

LEARNING OBJECTIVES

1. Understand groups as complex, open systems.
2. Apply the concept of open systems to healthcare teams.
3. Differentiate groups and teams.
4. Describe levels of systems and how they relate to healthcare teams.
5. Recognize how the diversity inherent to interprofessional healthcare teams contributes to their adaptability and sustainability.

Why Groups?

Humans are wired to be interdependent. We bond together in families, friendship groups, neighborhoods, work groups, and electronic social networks like Facebook and Twitter. The world has become more complex. The exponential growth of information that is required to solve problems is not the purview of a single person or a single profession. By recognizing our need to join with others to meet challenges, we have the opportunity for collective wisdom to emerge and facilitate the creation of new connections and innovative strategies to ensure the health and stability of the world that we share (Briskin et al., 2009). Groups and teams have been and will continue to be an essential part of our daily lives. Nowhere is the need for teamwork more relevant than in the healthcare arena.

Diagnosis and intervention require the efforts of a cadre of physician specialists, nurses, therapists, pharmacists, social services personnel, laboratory personnel, information managers, dietitians, transportation workers, home health aides, family caregivers, and patients. Quality health care that is accessible and cost effective requires that the boundaries between these stakeholders are made permeable through consistent collaboration (Schot et al., 2020). Skills in team building, team membership, and understanding group dynamics are foundational and indispensable for the next generation of healthcare leaders. Well-functioning healthcare teams are linked to good morale, reduced staff turnover, and positive patient outcomes (Gittell, 2009; Sampath et al., 2021; Dinh et al., 2020; Burtscher et al., 2020; Banerjee et al., 2016).

At our organization, everything is a committee decision. You can have input from multiple perspectives such as nursing, social work, occupational therapy, physical therapy, and dietary. Elder problems are highly complicated. Getting other perspectives is helpful. For example, let's say you can't transport Mrs. X into the center because she keeps hitting people and is not putting her seatbelt on. What do you do? You need to get different perspectives in order to make a decision. It is like that example of the blind men and the elephant. No single perspective will describe the elephant, and there probably is not one single resolution. This requires that team members are confident in what they know, amenable to listen to someone else's ideas, and willing to offer their own ideas.

—Karen J. Nichols, MD, Chief Medical Officer at Trinity Health PACE

What Distinguishes a Group from a Random Collection of People?

There is a unique designation for each of the myriad groupings in the animal kingdom, such as school (fish), troop (baboons), murder (crows), gam (whales), and group (humans). No matter what the species, the critical element that is common to all the groupings is that the individual members are interdependent. In the case of humans, "members are linked together in a web of interpersonal relationships. Thus, a group is defined as two or more individuals who are connected to one another by social relationships" (Forsyth, 2006, pp. 2–3). Alderfer (1977) expanded the definition of human groups to include how they are distinguished from and perceived by nonmembers and how they relate to other groups. For the purposes of this text, in order for a group to be distinguished from a random collection of people, its members must have common interests and goals and regular patterns of interaction, exert influence among the members, and work interdependently to achieve goals (Cartright & Zander, 1968; Lewin, 1948; Smith, 2008).

What Is the Difference Between a Team and a Group?

The terms *team* and *group* are often used interchangeably. However, making the distinction between these two terms can offer valuable insight into how groups work and can facilitate leadership and full participation in productive teams. The term *group* comes from the French word *groupe* and the Italian *gruppo*, which were borrowed originally from the prehistoric Germanic *kruppaz* and is translated into a "round mass, lump" (Online Etymology Dictionary, 2011). The term *group* is defined by Merriam-Webster (Definition of Group, 2011) as "a number of individuals assembled together or having some unifying relationship." *Team* is defined as a group that engages in more focused intentional action. The word is derived from the Middle English term *teme* and the Old English *tēon*, which is to draw or pull (Definition of Team, 2011). Katzenbach and Smith (1993) describe a team as "a small number of people with complementary skills who are committed to a common purpose, set of performance goals, and approach for which they hold themselves mutually accountable" (p. 112).

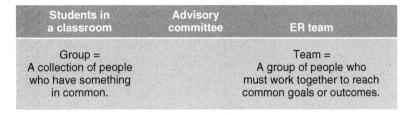

Students in a classroom	Advisory committee	ER team
Group = A collection of people who have something in common.		Team = A group of people who must work together to reach common goals or outcomes.

Figure 1.1 Group-team continuum.

REFLECTION: Identification of Groups

Rank in order the following descriptions with 1 being the most grouplike and 10 the least grouplike. Give reasons for your rankings.

_____ The spectators at a college football game
_____ Two strangers exchanging meaningful looks across a crowded bar
_____ A secretary conversing with the boss by telephone
_____ Five students at a university working together on a classroom assignment
_____ A mob of rioters burning stores in the inner city
_____ Thirteen inmates talking and lifting weights in a jail's exercise yard
_____ A committee deciding the best way to handle a production problem
_____ Six employees working on an assembly line
_____ An aggregate of individuals waiting in silence for a bus
_____ The Smith family of Richmond, Virginia (Mr. Smith, Mrs. Smith, and their daughter Jane Smith)

The difference between a group and a team can be described on a continuum (**Figure 1.1**). At one end of the spectrum, group refers to people with something in common and at the other end, team refers to people who must work together to get to a common agreed-upon goal or outcome. In this text, the term *group* will be used in discussions regarding the dynamics, processes, and patterns found in human collectives. Health professionals who are working together to achieve positive patient outcomes will be designated as *teams*.

A Systems Approach to Groups

Systems theory conceptualizes all physical and social systems as integrated wholes as opposed to agglomerations of disparate pieces.

The eighteenth-century German philosopher Hegel introduced systems theory by suggesting that the whole is more than the sum of its parts: the whole determines the nature of the parts and the parts are dynamically interrelated and cannot be understood in isolation from the whole. The biologist Ludwig von Bertanffly proposed that all biological systems are open to each other and each identifiable component is related to other parts (Banathy & Jenlink, 2004). From a systems theory perspective, an individual member of a team cannot fully be understood in isolation from the team, and a team cannot be fully understood without understanding the organizational context within which it exists.

Katz and Kahn (1978) explored the systems theory further when they proposed a method to analyze open (living) social systems. They posited that the interactive paradigm of analyzing living systems like organizations is based on continual cycles of input, throughput (processing), and outputs. All living organisms, like healthcare organizations and the groups that comprise them, are fully open systems. Some key characteristics of open systems resonate in the healthcare arena. Information provided by hospital staff, care recipients, suppliers, and funding sources is an example of input. Intervention from health professionals is an example of throughput, while patient outcomes, patient satisfaction rates, and quality improvement outcomes are examples of system outputs (Meyer & O'Brien-Pallas, 2010).

Healthcare organizations can be described as complex, adaptive systems because of the nonlinear and often unpredictable nature of the interactions among the many microsystems that compose the larger system (Sturmberg & Martin, 2013; Sampath et al., 2021). Suchman, Sluyter, and Williamson (2011) use the metaphor of a "gigantic complicated conversation" to describe the complex, open, nonlinear, and every evolving nature of healthcare organizations where the quality and quantity of systemic influence is dependent upon the nature of the interaction of all the constituencies within those organizations.

Each participant in a team takes in the ideas and opinions of others (input), processes this input and compares and integrates it with their most current thoughts (throughput), and together with the group, creates a new, collective perspective (output) (**Figure 1.2**) (Dinh et al., 2020). The organizational conversations reflect the organization's values, mission, culture, knowledge base, and interactive patterns among the microsystems/groups that compose the larger organization. Organizations that attempt to impose a mechanistic, linear orientation upon an inherently open system such as a group, organization, or community discount the value and challenges of randomness. These tightly coupled systems find themselves too rigid to respond

to internal or external signals for the need to change. For example, in a hierarchical healthcare system, team members are less likely to question designated leaders and are often unwilling or unable to be professionally assertive. As a result, the repertoire of solutions to problems may be limited and the team may be ill equipped to respond to change. Change in open systems is inevitable, and adapting to these environmental changes is a continuous process. The manner in which groups and their parent organizations respond to change determines the possibilities for or limits to creativity, productivity, and outcomes (Sturmberg & Martin, 2013; Sampath et al., 2021).

Systems, subsystems, and the environment are complex, interactive, and interdependent. The dynamic relationship between structure and function of all aspects of the system and its environment render the boundaries permeable, and changes at any level of a system affect all other levels of the system. For instance, organizational culture is as much a product of individual behaviors as it is a facilitator of individual behaviors (Studer, 2003). The mood of an individual leader can impact the mood of the team and be impacted by the tone of the team, or a team's effectiveness or ineffectiveness can impact and be impacted by the success of an organization (Edmondson, 2019). Nembhard and Edmondson (2006) found that inclusive behavior on the part of physician leaders yielded higher perceptions of psychological safety, increased engagement by all members of the healthcare team and concomitant positive quality improvement efforts. Healthcare organizations that have been able to institutionalize relationship building as a means for integrating myriad systems consistently report higher staff retention rates and better clinical outcomes (Gittell, 2009; Trzeciak et al., 2017).

Within all living systems, the balance between energy consumption (entropy) and

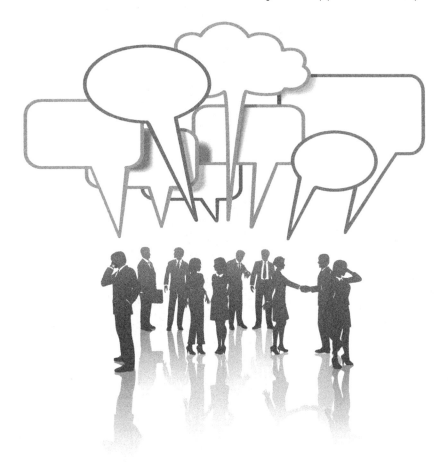

Figure 1.2 Conversations allow us to inquire, exchange and process information, expand thinking, and negotiate and transform that information into a common perspective that is different than the sum of its parts.

© Michael D. Brown/Shutterstock.

energy infusion (negentropy) is necessary for the maintenance of a steady state for optimal systems functioning (homeostasis). An example of this in healthcare practice is the effect of caretaker rest (energy infusion) on patient care (indicates status of system's functioning). The relationship between decreased caretaker rest and decreased cognitive and clinical performance on the part of the caretaker and concomitant medical errors has been well documented (Reed, Fletcher, & Arora, 2010).

The evolutionary capacity of a system depends on flexible and adaptable patterns of organization that facilitate its ability to deal with environmental challenges and opportunities. The most agile, adaptable, and successful healthcare teams are those that are able to routinely evaluate who needs to be present and who has the most cogent information or expertise (Nundy, 2021). Diverse perspectives and a broad range of information is essential for sound clinical decision-making (Briskin et al., 2009; Wheatley, 2005;

Burtscher et al., 2020). Inclusionary practices such as incorporating caregivers and support personnel into the healthcare team and giving equal attention to each team member's contribution broaden the perspective of the team. In addition, psychological safety and willingness of members to share information facilitates the generation of innovative solutions for improved patient care (Meyer & O'Brien-Pallas, 2010; Nembhard & Edmondson, 2006; Tannenbaum et al., 2021).

Applying Systems Theory

When attempting to study, understand, and effect change in a complex social system, it is helpful to distinguish among the individual, interpersonal, group, organizational, and community levels of the system.

Individual: One person.

Interpersonal: Two individuals interacting.

Group: Three or more individuals working toward a common goal or purpose.

Organization: A social structure, often made up of groups, that pursues a collective goal to deliver some product or service.

Community: Anything beyond the organizational level. This includes other organizations, governments, or global social networks.

Systematic analysis and intervention in complex organizations take the entire system into account (Rojas-Smith et al., 2014). Each interprofessional care team, department, or group can be considered a microsystem and can be examined with regard to its purpose, patients, professionals, processes, and patterns that distinguish it from and link it within the larger system. High-performing microsystems are characterized by inclusive leaders, strong organizational support, ongoing staff development, cohesive teams, patient/community focus, evidence-based practice, process improvement, and technology-enhanced communication through a variety of formal and informal channels (Barach & Johnson, 2006; Dinh et al., 2020; Tannenbaum et al., 2021).

Successful change agents, whether they are leaders or members of groups, learn to differentiate among systems levels, shift attention from one level to another, and make an informed decision about the best level at which to intervene based on a realistic appraisal of the change agent's sphere of influence (Wells, 1995). Sturmber and Martin (2013) contend that intervention in complex systems is most effective when problem solvers consider the system from a variety of perspectives, frequently test hypotheses, engage in structured problem solving, practice self-reflection, and consider goals in light of their effects on the whole system (Schot, 2019). While the primary focus of this text is the group level of system, individual and interpersonal levels will also be explored. **Table 1.1** shows examples of intervention methods that are commonly used at various system levels.

Our current healthcare system is one that is complex and changing rapidly. It can been described as volatile, uncertain, complex, and ambiguous or VUCA. VUCA is a concept that was originally developed by the military and has since been applied to the rapidly evolving healthcare environment. Using a systems perspective helps to address the challenges of a VUCA world by engaging all stakeholders in conversations that will leverage their expertise and resources, broaden and strengthen relationships among stakeholders, engender creative problem solving, and inspire the diffusion of new ideas and practices (Sturmberg & Martin, 2013; Lindberg et al., 2013; Edmonson, 2019; Weber, 2013).

Table 1.1 Intervention at Each Level of System

Level	Focus	Goal	Methods
Individual	Individual's behavior, perceptions, and emotions	Increase self-awareness and self-management	Coaching, training, mentoring, and feedback
Interpersonal	The relationship and communication between two people	Clarify the nature of the relationship and goals and strengthen foundations for clear communication	Conflict management, mediation, communication, and conflict resolution training
Group	Group goals, tasks, roles	Clarify the nature of individual contributions, the group's purpose, and group behaviors that will foster accomplishment of goals	Education and feedback on the stages of group development, team building, leadership, and coaching behaviors that contribute to team effectiveness and productivity
Organization	Culture, leadership development, and organizational strategy and structure	Increase awareness of the people in the organization that the whole is different from the sum of its parts; identify what attributes, behaviors, and strategies are necessary in order to reach the organizational goals	Analysis of organizational state including culture, training in culture change, top team development, and executive coaching; identify organizational strengths in order to leverage culture change, appreciative inquiry, and dynamic inquiry
Community	Finding common ground so that the community can be served	Building partnerships and collaborations across communities to deliver services	Strategic planning, community development, and futuring

CASE STUDY   **System-Level Intervention**

The chair of the pediatrics department in a large health system, Dr. Clarice Barna was struggling with a problem. Three of the 75 residents asked for a meeting with her. During the meeting, the residents complained that they were getting inconsistent instruction from the faculty and not getting the feedback and one-on-one attention from the faculty they felt they deserved. They also felt that the nurses often gave them different instructions than the ones they got from the faculty about patient care. Although three residents were in

the meeting, almost all of the talking was done by one resident, Jason.

Dr. Barna set up a meeting with the faculty and shared Jason's feedback on behalf of the residents. The faculty discussed ways to improve instruction and thought that it would be good to get additional feedback from the nurses. The faculty expressed frustration that the residents, although great students, seemed to get confused when trying to grasp that there can be more than one way to do a procedure. Each of the faculty had unique

(continues)

perspectives and practices they wanted to offer the residents and felt the residents needed to understand and accept multiple methods for procedures.

Dr. Barna then discussed the situation with the nursing team that worked most often with the residents. The nurses said they really enjoyed working with the residents and that they were really a top-notch group. The head nurse, Eileen Fenway, upon hearing that Jason was the student who brought this up, reminded the chair that Jason completed his internship at University Children's Hospital where the interns were each assigned a specific mentor, coach, and technical instructor in addition to

faculty. She suggested that Jason's perception and expectations needed to be addressed.

Questions:

1. Look at the row labeled "Individual" in Table 1.1. Assume that Jason is the individual. Describe how Dr. Barna could improve things by talking only to Jason.
2. Look at the row labeled "Group" in Table 1.1. Describe how Dr. Barna could engage the group of faculty and nurses to help achieve the goals of improving resident education based on the feedback given by the residents.

References

Alderfer, C. P. (1977). Organization development. *Annual Review of Psychology, 28,* 197–223.

Banathy, B. H., & Jenlink, P. M. (2004). Systems inquiry and its application in education. In D. H. Jonassen (Ed.), *Handbook of research on educational communications and technology* (pp. 37–57). Lawrence Erlbaum Associates.

Banerjee, A., Slagle, J., Mercalso, N., Booker, R., Miller, A., France, D., Rawn, L., & Weinger, M. (2016). A simulation–based curriculum to introduce key teamwork principles to entering medical students. *BMC Medical Education 16,* 295. DOI 10.1186/s12909-016-0808-9

Barach, P., & Johnson, J. (2006). Understanding the complexity of redesigning care around the clinical microsystem. *Quality & Safety in Healthcare, 15*(Suppl I): i10–i16.

Briskin, A., Erickson, S., Ott, J., & Callanan, T. (2009). *The power of collective wisdom and the trap of collective folly.* San Francisco, CA: Berrett-Koehler.

Burtscher, M. J., Nussbeck, F. W., Sevdalis, N., Gisin, S., & Manser, T. (2020). Coordination and communication in healthcare action teams: The role of expertise. *Swiss Journal of Psychology, 79*(3–4), 123–135. https://doi.org/10.1024/1421-0185/a000239

Cartright, D., & Zander, A. (1968). *Group dynamics: Research and theory.* Harper & Row Publishers.

Definition of Group. (2011). *Merriam-webster.com.* http://www.merriam-webster.com/dictionary/group

Definition of Team. (2016). *Merriam-webster.com.* http://www.merriam-webster.com/dictionary/team

Dinh, J., Traylor, A., Kilcullen, M., Perez, J., Scheweissing, E., Venkatesh, A. & Salas, E. (2020). Cross disciplinary care: A systematic review on teamwork processes in health care. *Small Group Research, 51*(1), 125–166. doi: 10.1177/1046496419872002

Edmondson, A. (2019). *The fearless organization: creating psychological safety in the work place for learning, innovation and growth.* Wiley & Sons.

Forsyth, D. R. (2006). *Group dynamics* (4th ed. [International student edition.]). Thomson Wadsworth Publishing.

Gittell, J. (2009). *High performance healthcare: Using the power of relationships to achieve quality, efficiency and resilience.* McGraw-Hill.

Katz, D., & Kahn, R. (1978). *The social psychology of organizations.* Wiley.

Katzenbach, J. R., & Smith, D. K. (1993). *The wisdom of teams: Creating the high-performance organization.* Harvard Business School.

Lewin, K., & Lewin, G. W. (Eds.). (1948). *Resolving social conflicts: Selected papers on group dynamics.* Harper & Row.

Lindberg, C., Hatch, M., Mohl, V., Arce, C., & Ciemins, E. (2013). Embracing uncertainty: Complexity-inspired innovations at Billings Clinic. In J. Sturmberg & C. Martin (Eds.), *Handbook of systems and complexity in health* (pp. 697–713). Springer Science + Business Media.

Online Etymology Dictionary. (2016). group.*Etymonline.com.* http://www.etymonline.com/index.php?allowed_in_frame=0&search=group

Meyer, R. M., & O'Brien-Pallas, L. L. (2010). Nursing services delivery theory: An open system approach. *Journal of Advanced Nursing, 66*(12), 2828–2838.

Nembhard, I., & Edmondson, A. (2006). Making it safe: The effects of leader inclusiveness and professional status on psychological safety and improvement efforts in health care teams. *Journal of Organizational Behavior, 27*, 941–966.

Nundy, S. (2021). *Care after COVID: What the pandemic revealed is broken in healthcare and how to reinvent it.* McGraw Hill.

Reed, D., Fletcher, K., & Arora, V. (2010). Systemic review: Association of shift length, protected sleep time and night float with patient care, residents' health and education. *Annals of Internal Medicine, 53*, 829–842.

Rojas-Smith, L., Ashok, M., & Morss-Dy, S. (2014). *Contextual frameworks for research on the implementation of complex system interventions (internet).* Agency for Healthcare Research and Quality.

Sampath, B., Rakover, J., Baldoza, K., Mate, K., Lenoci-Edwards, j., & Barker, P. (2021). *Whole system quality: A unified approach to building responsive, resilient health care systems.* IHI White Paper. Institute for Healthcare Improvement.

Schot, E., Tummers, L., & Noordegraaf, M. (2020). Working on working together. A systematic review on how healthcare professionals contribute to interprofessional collaboration. *Journal of Interprofessional Care, 34*(3), 332–342, DOI: 10.1080/13561820.2019.1636007

Smith, M. (2008). *Experience in groups and other papers.* Tavistock Publications Limited.

Studer, Q. (2003). *Hardwiring excellence: Purpose, worthwhile work, making a difference.* Fire Starter Publishing.

Sturmberg, J., & Martin, C. (Eds.). (2013). Complexity in health: An introduction. In J. Sturmberg & C. Martin (Eds.), *Handbook of systems and complexity in health* (pp. 1–17). Springer Science + Business Media.

Suchman, A., Sluyter, D., & Williamson, P. (2011). *Leading change in healthcare: Transforming organizations using complexity, positive psychology and relationship-centered care.* Radcliffe Publishing.

Tannenbaum, S., Traylor, A., Thomas, E., & Salas, E. (2021). Managing teamwork in the face of a pandemic: evidence based tips. *BMJ Quality & Safety, 30*, 59–63.

Torrens, P. (2010). The health care team members: Who are they and what do they do? In B. Freshman, L. Rubino, & Y. Chassiakos (Eds.), *Collaboration across the disciplines in health care* (pp. 1–19). Jones and Bartlett Publishers.

Trezeciak, S., Roberts, B., & Mazzerelli, A. (2017). *Compassionomics: Hypothesis and experimental approach.* Cooper University Health care and Cooper Medical School of Rowan University.

Weber, C. (2013). *Conversational capacity: The secret to building successful teams that perform when the pressure is on.* McGraw Hill.

Wells, L. (1995). The group as a whole: A systemic socio-analytic perspective on interpersonal and group relations. In G. Gillette, & M. McCollum (Eds.), *Groups in context* (pp. 50–85). Lanham, MD: University Press of America.

Wheatley, M. (2005). *Finding our way: Leadership for an uncertain time.* Berret-Koehler Publishers, Inc.

CHAPTER 2

Group Development

LEARNING OBJECTIVES

1. Discuss aspects of small group behavior theory as described in the literature.
2. Examine the conscious and unconscious components of group life.
3. Differentiate between the developmental stages of group life.
4. Analyze group behavior.
5. Facilitate teamwork throughout the group life-span.

The Group

As members or leaders of groups, most of us notice the personalities of the members of the group, the topics discussed, the disagreements, and our own emotions. While individualistic Western cultures routinely view groups as collections of individuals, Eastern cultures have long recognized groups as distinct collectives rather than a collection of distinct individuals (Hofstede, 1983) (**Figure 2.1**).

This perspective informs the way the group harnesses its power in order to get something done. Shifting from an *I* perspective to a *We* perspective recognizes the group as a source of intelligence that is greater than any one individual. The *We* perspective facilitates the integration, engagement, and creation of collective wisdom—ultimately achieving a whole that is more powerful and creative than the sum of its parts (Briskin et al., 2009).

All groups demonstrate consistent patterns of member, leader, and group behaviors as they relate to the acquisition of roles, the assumption of and response to authority, norm development, and communication patterns. These patterns serve as indicators of developmental changes in the group over time. Neuroscience supports the notion of a social brain—a neurophysiological conduit for perceiving, processing, and mirroring the emotions and behaviors of others. In other words, our interactions with each other in groups have the potential to trigger neuronal activity, which, in turn, influences our emotions and behaviors (Goleman, 2011). Positive or negative action on the part of one person can trigger a like reaction in another. When repeated often enough, this positive or negative interaction pattern becomes a group norm (Frederickson, 2003).

We have all experienced a time when we were in sync or on the same wavelength or

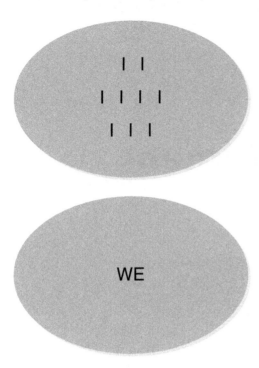

Figure 2.1 The I/We perception.

connected with another individual or group of individuals on a level that transcended the social psychological aspects of engagement. Integrating the systemic laws of neuropsychology and physics with social psychology, Rene Levi (2005) examined and labeled these transcendent experiences as "collective resonance" and defined it as follows:

> A felt sense of energy, rhythm, or intuitive knowing that occurs in a group of human beings and positively affects the way they interact toward a positive purpose . . . that enables us to make greater progress toward our common human goals than we have been able to do using idea exchange and analytic problem-solving alone. (p. 1)

This view is consistent with the "Weness" inherent to the Eastern conceptualization of groups and the emergence of collective intelligence in collectives of all types—including teams,

organizations, and communities. It is important to note that these potentially generative, interactive, and integrative tendencies are inherent to humans and, when not managed mindfully, can devolve into group dysfunction or what Briskin et al. (2009) refer to as "collective folly." In these instances, the focus is on the barriers that divide and polarize the group rather than the connections that unify it (Briskin et al., 2009).

These interactive patterns, carried out over the life of the group, contribute to the development of a unique social organism that is more than the sum of its parts (Bion, 1974; Lewin, 1951; Perls et al., 1951; Tilin & Broder, 2005; Tuckman, 1965; Wheelan, 2005).

Each of the columns in **Table 2.1** represents a level of system in group life—the individual members within the group, the group as a unit, and the context or the environment within which the group exists. Under each component are aspects that contribute to the social-psychological landscape of every group at any point in time. The study of group dynamics attempts to analyze and interpret group life by examining these aspects in a systematic fashion.

What You See Is Not What You Get: The Unconscious Life of a Group

Wilfred Bion, a psychoanalyst, was one of the first researchers to identify patterns in groups. Bion maintained that groups have a conscious and an unconscious life. He named the conscious group the *work group* and the unconscious group the *basic assumption group*. The conscious work group focuses on rationally accomplishing overt tasks and activities. The basic assumption group describes the unconscious aspects of a group. Leaders and members often mistakenly perceive these unconscious aspects as interfering with the real work of the group. In fact, this is the way that the collective membership and leadership of

Table 2.1 Levels of the System in Group Life

Behavior—How does each member behave in the group?	**Norms/rules**—What are the explicit/tacit rules for behavior in this group?	**Physical/social proximity**—How much time does the group spend together?
Personal feelings—How do each of the members feel about working in the group?	**Roles**—Who are the talkers/listeners?	**Relations with outsiders**—Which are stronger, members' intragroup or extragroup relations?
Internalized norms—What are the personal rules that are held by each member?	**Authority**—Who are the leaders/followers?	**Responsibilities/expectations**—What is expected of this group?
Beliefs/values—What beliefs/values influence each member?	**Communication**—Who talks to whom?	**Cultural issues**—What are the cultural issues (age, ethnic, gender, professional) that might affect this group?
Self-concept—How does each member see himself or herself functioning in the group?		**Level of autonomy**—How much control over the outcomes of this group does the group have?

the group deal with the anxiety and polarities of individual identity and collective identity. Bion specifically identified the following three basic assumptions: dependency, fight-flight, and pairing (**Table 2.2**). Leaders and members who learn to identify these group processes as a natural part of a group's development are better prepared to be positive catalysts in the group. Rather than being caught up in the anxiety of the group, this knowledge can allow a person to be more objective, emotionally independent, and prepared to act in a constructive manner (Bennis & Shepherd, 1956, pp. 417–418).

Stages of Group Development

While multiple factors influence group functioning, each group—like each human being—should be considered a unique organism that passes through predictable phases of development. Characteristic member, leader, and group behaviors, as they relate to the acquisition of roles, the assumption of and response to authority, norm development, and communication patterns—like human developmental milestones—serve as

indicators of developmental changes in the group over time. Awareness of the interacting determinants of group behavior and the unconscious assumptions of the group will facilitate an understanding of group behavior and facilitate effective group leadership and participation.

Groups display behavioral patterns that are common to all groups and are not dependent on the individuals in the group. A number of theorists have used various terms to describe the key issues that groups address over their life-span. While these issues are ever present, some issues gain primacy, depending upon the developmental level of the group. In summary, the group, as a whole, struggles to find the right balance between the unconscious desire to have a group identity and retain individual identities. Over time, a group is also challenged with dealing with the paradox of being safely protected by an omnipotent leader and taking control of its own destiny. A mature group learns to deal effectively with these issues. Its members work cooperatively as separate and discrete members who willingly choose to belong to the group because they identify with interests of the group. This

Table 2.2 Wilfred Bion Summary

	Group Aim	Anxiety	Member	Leader	Behavior
Unconscious Dependency	Security	Anxiety is reduced through leader's superhuman ability to care for the group.	Knows nothing, inadequate, and childlike.	Omnipotent, parent, and protector.	Leader makes all decisions, provides all direction, and solves all problems.
Fight or flight	Balance group identity with individual identities	Anxiety is expressed by resisting or fleeing the group dynamic.	Paradoxically struggles to balance group identity with personal identity.	Leader loses omnipotent status and is often blamed for not resolving the individual versus group problem.	Fluctuates between arguing and avoiding difficult topics. Scapegoating: Individuals and leaders can be sacrificed for the sake of the group.
Pairing	Hope and optimism	Anxiety is reduced by letting the pair take control.	Let the pair do the work.	The pair acts on behalf of the leader.	Two people in the group take on the task of working out the unconscious group dilemmas.
Conscious Work group	Fulfills the actual goals and tasks of a group	Anxiety is reduced enough to focus on work.	Contributes to the group reaching its goals.	Contributes to the group reaching its goals.	Leader members will support the group to achieve tangible goals.

Data from Bion, W. (1974). *Experiences in groups: And other papers.* Science and Behavior Books.

group tests its conclusions, seeks knowledge, learns from its experience, and is in agreement with regard to the group's purpose and tasks (Bales, 1950; Bion, 1974; Rioch, 1983; Schutz, 1958; Tuckman, 1965; Wheelan, 2005; Yalom, 1995).

Tuckman (1965) conducted an extensive review of the group development literature and concluded that therapy groups, work groups, and human relations training groups (t-groups) had strong developmental similarities despite differences in group composition, task, goal, and the duration of group life. He noted a few critical common themes about groups:

- There is a distinction between groups as a social entity and a task entity.
- In all groups, the task and the social emotional functions occur simultaneously.
- All groups go through four stages of group development. The task and

social-emotional functions are different for each stage.

- The group moves from one stage to the next by successfully accomplishing the task and social-emotional/group structure function at each stage.

Tuckman named these stages of group development *forming*, *storming*, *norming*, and *performing* (**Table 2.3**). He later added a fifth stage called *adjourning*, which describes the characteristics of groups as they terminate.

An Integrated Model of Group Development

Susan Wheelan (2005) used empirical research to build on Tuckman's model. She proposed and validated an integrated model of group development using the Group Development

Table 2.3 Tuckman's Description of the Stages of Group Development Based on Literature Review of Therapy and T-Groups

	Task Issues	Structure and Social-Emotional Issues
Forming	**Orientation to the task:** Group members attempt to define the group task by identifying information that will be needed and the ground rules that must be followed to complete the job of the group.	**Testing and dependence:** Group members attempt to discover acceptable behavior according to the leader and other group members.
Storming	**Emotional response to task demands:** Group members act emotionally to task demands and exhibit resistance to suggested actions.	**Intragroup conflict:** Group members disagree with one another and the leader as a way to express their own individuality.
Norming	**Discussing oneself and others:** Group members listen to each other and the leader and use information and input from everyone.	**Development of group cohesion:** Group members accept the group and the individuality of fellow members, thus becoming an entity through rule agreement and role clarification.
Performing	**Emergence of insight:** A variety of methods of inquiry are used and members adjust their behavior to serve the greater goals of the group.	**Functional role relatedness:** Members are focused on getting the task done and relate to each other in ways that will accomplish the task.

Data from Tuckman, B. (1965). Developmental sequence in small groups. *Psychological Bulletin, 63*(6), 384–394.

Questionnaire (GDQ) (Wheelan, 1990; Wheelan & Hochberger, 1996). Using observational and survey data, this integrated model is consistent with previous models in that it describes group stages developing naturally and in a chronological fashion over time. In addition, Wheelan and her team of researchers found the following:

- Specific characteristics emerge in each stage of a group's development. Early stages of group development are associated with specific issues and patterns of speech, such as those related to dependency, counter-dependency, and trust, which precede the actual work conducted during the more mature stages of a group's life.
- Groups navigate through the stages by accomplishing process-oriented goals like achieving a certain degree of member safety, expressing and tolerating different opinions, and devising agreed-upon methods of decision-making.
- Most groups need a normative time frame in order to traverse each stage.
- Organizational culture influences group norms and can influence group development.

- Member and leader behaviors are equally important in the development of a group, and the dynamic between them must be addressed as the group develops.

Identifying the Stages of Group Development: Characteristics and Goals

While stages of group development are identified by the issues that predominate, a percentage of group energy is always expended on dependency, conflict, trust, and work regardless of the stage (**Figure 2.2**). For example, work gets done at every stage of development. In earlier stages, most of the work is done under the leader's direction. In succeeding stages, members take increasingly more responsibility. By Stages III and IV, responsibility for work is evenly distributed among the members, and the leader is used as a resource. The key challenge for group members and leaders is finding

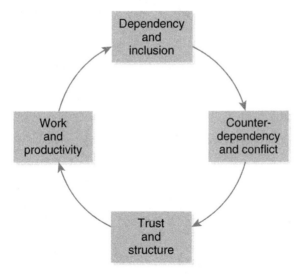

Figure 2.2 Key developmental issues of group life.

Data from Wheelan, S. (2005). *Group processes: A developmental perspective* (2nd ed.). Allyn and Bacon.

the balance between task and social-emotional issues and managing the conflict that these issues engender over the life-span of the group. Wheelan and Williams (2003) found that the communication content of groups over their life-span mirror key developmental issues (**Table 2.4**). In other words, the amount of time spent talking about task-related concerns increases over the life of the group, while the amount of time talking about social-emotional concerns decreases as the group matures. **Figures 2.3A, B,** and **C** provide an example

of how the proportion of attention on key issues might shift based on the developmental level of the group. As with people, no one size fits all and each group ultimately demonstrates unique developmental patterns.

Stage I (Dependency/Inclusion) is characterized by significant member dependency on the designated leader, concerns about safety, and inclusion issues. In this stage, members rely on the leader and powerful group members to provide direction. This is manifested by the percentage of statements that address

Table 2.4 Wheelan: An Integrated Model of Group Development

I: Dependency/Inclusion	▪ Tentative and polite ▪ High compliance ▪ Rarely express disagreement ▪ Fear rejection ▪ Conflict limited ▪ Conformity high	▪ Assumes consensus ▪ Roles based on external status and first impressions ▪ Communication centralized ▪ Lacks structure and organization	▪ Seen as benevolent and competent ▪ Is expected to provide direction and safety ▪ Is rarely challenged ▪ Leader should facilitate communications, safety, and set standards
II: Counterdependency/Conflict	▪ Disagree about goals and tasks ▪ Feel safer to dissent ▪ Challenge the leader ▪ Increase participation	▪ Conflicts emerge ▪ Goal and role clarification begins ▪ Decreasing conformity ▪ Subgroups form ▪ Intolerance for subgroups ▪ Conflict management attempted ▪ Successful conflict resolution increases consensus (i.e., goals) and culture ▪ Trust and cohesion increases	▪ Is challenged frequently ▪ Leader should help develop values, accept changes, and encourage independence
III: Trust/Structure	▪ Satisfaction increases ▪ Commitment to group tasks is high	▪ Increased goal clarity and consensus ▪ Communications structure more flexible ▪ Communications content more task oriented	▪ Leaders should be less directive, egalitarian, and more consultative

(continues)

Table 2.4 Wheelan: An Integrated Model of Group Development   *(continued)*

IV: Work/Productivity		
■ Clear about group goals ■ Agree with group goals ■ Clear about their roles ■ Voluntary conformity is high ■ Cooperative	■ Role assignments match member abilities ■ Communications structure matches task demands ■ Open communication allows participation of all members ■ Receives, gives, and uses feedback ■ Plans how to solve problems and make decisions ■ Implements and evaluates solutions and decisions ■ Highly cohesive ■ Task-related deviances tolerated	■ Style matches group developmental level ■ Delegates ■ Leaders should move toward nonleadership

dependency and pairing (when two people couple or pair by giving mutual compliments to each other) (8 percent and 16 percent, respectively). Statements regarding conflict are few (about 6 percent). About 17 percent of the time, team members engage in safe, noncontroversial discussions filled with flight statements by exchanging stories about outside activities or other topics that are not relevant to group goals while approximately 50 percent of the time is spent on work-related issues. The goals at Stage I are to create a sense of belonging and the beginnings of predictable patterns of interaction, develop member

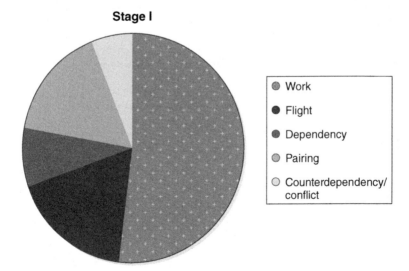

Stage I

Legend:
- Work
- Flight
- Dependency
- Pairing
- Counterdependency/conflict

Figure 2.3A Stage I.

Data from Wheelan S. (2005). *Group processes: A developmental perspective* (2nd ed.). Allyn and Bacon.

Stage II

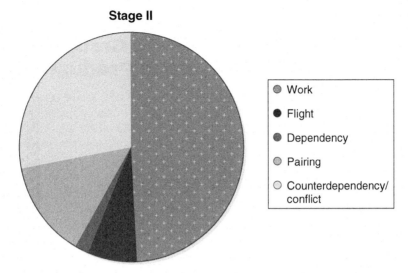

Figure 2.3B Stage II.

Data from Wheelan, S. (2005). *Group processes: A developmental perspective* (2nd ed.). Allyn and Bacon.

Stage III/IV

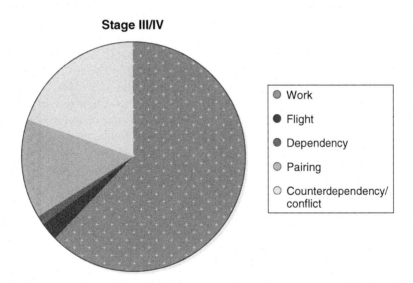

Figure 2.3C Stage III/IV.

Data from Wheelan, S. (2005). *Group processes: A developmental perspective* (2nd ed.). Allyn and Bacon.

loyalty to the group, and create an environment in which members feel safe enough to contribute ideas and suggestions.

Stage II (Counterdependency/Conflict) is characterized by member disagreement about group goals and procedures. Conflict is inevitable. Flight statements decrease to about 7 percent and work statements remain at 49 percent. Dependency statements fall to 2 percent, and those regarding conflict rise to 28 percent. Expressing disagreements and working them out is a necessary part of this process and allows members to communicate and begin to establish a trusting climate in which members feel free to disagree with each other and collaborate. The goals for Stage II are to develop a unified set of goals, values, and operational procedures, and to strike a balance between respect for the individual contributions and mediating individual needs with the group needs.

Stage III (Trust/Structure) is characterized by more mature negotiations about roles, organization, and procedures. The primary goal for Stage III is to solidify positive relationships that benefit the productivity of the group.

Stage IV (Work/Productivity) is characterized by a time of intense team productivity and effectiveness. Having resolved many of the issues of the previous stages, the group can focus most of its energy on goal achievement and task accomplishment. Roughly 62 percent of statements are related to work, and 20 percent of the time is spent on sorting out differences of opinion on how the work should get done. At this point the group is resilient enough to remain cohesive while encouraging task-related conflicts.

Termination: When groups face their own ending point, some may address separation issues and members' appreciation of each other and the group experience. In other groups the impending end may cause disruption and conflict.

REFLECTION: Identify the Stage of a Group

Which stage does the behavior indicate?

- Members are listening and seeking to understand one another.
- Members attempt to figure out their roles and functions.
- Divisive feelings and subgroups within the group increase.
- Group members follow a self-appointed or designated leader's suggestions without enthusiasm.
- Disagreements become more civilized and less angry and emotional.
- Members argue with one another, even when they agree on the basic issues.

How Does the Stage of the Group Impact Team Productivity?

Wheelan (2005) found that aspects such as group size and group age affect development and productivity. It usually takes at least 6 months for a group to achieve the Stage IV developmental level. Newly formed groups are characterized by a higher percentage of dependency and counterdependency/flight statements ("I don't know what to do." "The leader is incompetent." "Did you see the game last night?"), while more established groups make more work statements ("Let's focus on the task at hand."). These findings are corroborated by Nembhard and Edmondson (2006), who found that long-standing membership in healthcare teams was correlated with the willingness of all members, irrespective of status, to share information and provide innovative solutions—behaviors that are indicative of more mature groups.

In a study involving 17 intensive care units, Wheelan, Davidson, and Tilin (2003) found a link between perceived group maturity and patients' outcomes in intensive care units. Staff members of units with mortality rates that were lower than predicted perceived their teams as functioning at higher stages of group development. They perceived their team members as less dependent and more trusting than did staff members of units with mortality rates that were higher than predicted. Staff members of high-performing units also perceived their teams as more structured and organized than did staff members of lower performing units.

Group Size: Less Is More

It is not uncommon to hear members of groups complain that some members of the group are doing more work than others. This perceptual phenomenon can happen in any sized group, but studies show that the larger the group, the less energy any individual exerts. In the late-nineteenth century, Maximillian Ringelman performed one of the first experiments with group size by having groups of people play tug of war. He discovered that as the total number of people who pulled the rope increased, the less each individual contributed. Ringelman called this phenomenon "social loafing." In addition, larger groups tend to have a more difficult time coalescing around a single identity and distributing work in an equitable fashion. Studies indicate that cohesion and intimacy decrease as team size increases (Bogart & Lundgren, 1974; Fisher, 1953;

Seashore, 1954). Members of larger groups perceive their groups to be more competitive, less cohesive, more argumentative, and less satisfying (Steiner, 1972). Wheelan (2009) found that small groups tended to be more productive than large groups, and small groups reached mature levels of group development more rapidly than large groups (**Figure 2.4**).

The literature seems to indicate that groups are most productive when they are composed of three to eight members. Theoretically, this is because the larger the group, the longer and more difficult it is for the group to develop a common identity.

CASE STORY **How Many People Are Needed to Make This Decision?**

Our team needs to make decisions regarding who should be enrolled in the program. Some applications could potentially be denied for various reasons. When I first got here, 40 people were in the morning meeting where these decisions were made. Everyone read the report at that meeting, and after the coffee kicked in, people were talking amongst themselves, others were listening, and others were on cell phones. People were just getting confused, and the decision process was taking around 2 hours. I worked with the marketing people and changed this system. We now have a separate

smaller group of eight people in a meeting that includes social work, nursing, a physician, and transportation; four marketing people give input but don't get a vote. We invite additional guests from other departments, such as behavioral medicine as needed.

At first, a lot of stress was associated with the transition because change is stressful. But after 6 months, the length of time from intake to decision was cut dramatically. The morning meeting can be done in 15 minutes!

—Karen J. Nichols, MD, Chief Medical Officer at Trinity Health PACE

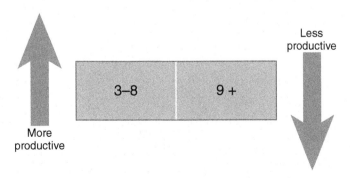

Figure 2.4 Correlation of group size and productivity. According to Wheelan, groups of three to eight were more productive and more mature at 6 months than groups with nine or more members.

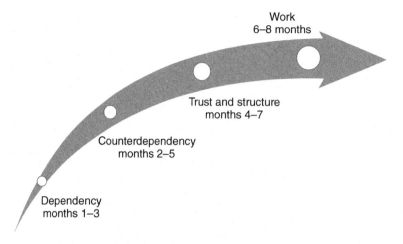

Figure 2.5 Time it takes for groups to mature.

Modified from Wheelan, S., Davidson, B., & Tilin, F. (2003). Group development across time: reality or illusion? *Small Group Research, 34*(2), 223–245.

How Long Does It Take for a Group to Develop Through Each Stage?

Research suggests that it takes time for groups to mature (Wheelan, Davidson, & Tilin, 2003). Under the right circumstances, intact groups or groups that have unchanging membership, can reach full maturity in 6 to 8 months. Shifting membership is commonplace in healthcare teams and presents challenges to group development and team coordination and performance. The ability to adapt to these changes is of paramount importance. Training in teamwork skills, efficient and effective communication sharing, and rotating leadership based on expertise mitigates the challenges to group development created by shifting membership (Bedwell et al., 2012; Interprofessional Education Collaborative, 2016; Schot et al., 2020).

Figure 2.5 is meant to be a guide to the average amount of time researchers have ascribed to the stages of development based on the integrated model of group development. Every group is a bit different, and some may actually get stuck at a certain level of development and take longer to move on to the next stage. Issues such as fluidity of membership, culture, diversity, group management, organizational dynamics, and complexity of tasks, as well as group commitment and identity impact the way groups develop and how well they perform.

References

Bales, R. (1950). *Interaction process analysis: A method for the study of small groups.* Addison-Wesley.

Bedwell, W., Ramsay, S., & Salas, E. (2012). Helping fluid teams work: A research agenda for effective team adaptation in healthcare. *Translational Behavioral Medicine, 2,* 504–509. doi 10.1007/s13142—12-0177-9

Bennis, W. G., & Shepherd, H. A. (1956). A theory of group development. *Human Relations, 9,* 415–437.

Bion, W. (1974). *Experiences in groups: And other papers.* Science and Behavior Books.

Bogart, D., & Lundgren, D. (1974). Group size, member dissatisfaction, and group radicalism. *Human Relations, 27*(4), 339–355.

Briskin, A., Erickson, S., Ott, J., & Callanan, T. (2009). *The power of collective wisdom and the trap of collective folly.* Berrett-Koehler.

Fisher, P. H. (1953). An analysis of the primary group. *Sociometry, 16,* 272–276.

Frederickson, B. (2003). The value of positive emotions. *American Scientist, 91,* 330–335.

Goleman, D. (2011). *Leadership: The power of emotional intelligence.* More Than Sound.

Hofstede, G. (1983). The cultural relativity of organizational practices and theories. *Journal of International Business Studies, 14*(2), 75–89.

Interprofessional Education Collaborative. (2016). *Core competencies for interprofessional collaborative practice: 2016 Update.* Interprofessional Education Collaborative.

Levi, R. (2005). What is resonance? *The Resonance Project.* http://resonanceproject.org/welcome1.cfm?pt=0&id=73

Lewin, K. (1951). *Field theory in social science.* Harper and Row.

Nembhard, I., & Edmondson, A. (2006). Making it safe: The effects of leader inclusiveness and professional status on psychological safety and improvement efforts in health care teams. *Journal of Organizational Behavior, 27,* 941–966.

Perls, F., Hefferline, R., & Goodman, P. (1951). *Gestalt therapy: Excitement and growth in the human personality.* Julian Press.

Rioch, M. J. (1983). The work of Wilfred Bion in groups. In A. Coleman & W. H. Bexron (Eds.). *Group relations reader 1* (pp. 21–32). A.K. Rice Institute Series.

Schot, E., Tummers, L., & Noordegraaf, M. (2020). Working on working together. A systematic review on how healthcare professionals contribute to interprofessional collaboration. *Journal of Interprofessional Care, 34*(3), 332–342, doi: 10.1080/13561820.2019.1636007

Schutz, W. (1958). *FIRO: A three dimensional theory of interpersonal behavior.* Rinehart.

Seashore, S. (1954). *Group cohesiveness in the industrial work group.* Institute for Social Research.

Steiner, I. (1972). *Group process and productivity.* Academic Press.

Tilin, F., & Broder, J. (2005). Team consultation. In S. A. Wheelan (Ed.), *The handbook of group research and practice* (pp. 427–439). Sage Publications.

Tuckman, B. (1965). Developmental sequence in small groups. *Psychological Bulletin, 63*(6), 384–394.

Wheelan, S. (1990). *Facilitating training groups: A guide to leadership and verbal intervention skills.* Praeger.

Wheelan, S. (2005). *Group process: A developmental perspective* (2nd ed.). Allyn & Bacon.

Wheelan, S., Davidson, B., & Tilin, F. (2003). Group development across time: Reality or illusion? *Small Group Research, 34*(2), 223–245.

Wheelan, S., & Hochberger, J. (1996). Validation studies of the group development questionnaire. *Small Group Research, 27*(1), 143–170.

Wheelan, S. A., & Williams, T. (2003). Mapping dynamic interaction patterns in work groups. *Small Group Research, 34*(4), 443–467. https://doi.org/10.1177/1046496403254043

Wheelan, S. A. (2009). Group size, group development, and productivity. *Small Group Research, 40*(2), 247–262.

Yalom, I. (1995). *The theory and practice of group psychotherapy* (4th ed.). Basic Books.

© oxygen/Moment/Getty Images

Team Building Blocks: Norms, Goals, Roles, Communication, Leaders, and Members

LEARNING OBJECTIVES

1. Explore how personality, environment, goals, roles, and communication impact group development.
2. Differentiate personal and group needs.
3. Recognize how norms shape team behavior.
4. Understand the value of giving and receiving feedback.
5. Match communication style to the needs of the listener.

Norms

Group norms are agreed-upon standards of behavior. Norms are the shared explicit or implicit rules that a group uses to identify standards of performance and distinguish appropriate from inappropriate behavior. When group norms are explicit or made explicit, they are commonly referred to as ground rules, agreements, group charters, conditions, or guidelines. However, not all norms are explicit, and the perceptions and concomitant behavior of individuals in groups is profoundly—and often unconsciously—affected by social influence (Sherif, 1936).

In many progressive organizations, errors are considered teaching moments that provide opportunities for open discussion, team-based problem-solving, and continuous improvement. In health care, the dire consequences of medical mistakes tend to discourage the very discussions of errors that are necessary to prevent their occurrence (O'Daniel & Rosenstein, 2008). This tendency, in combination with differing professional identities, cultures, skills, domains of concern, differences in power, capacity, resources, goals, and accountability actually requires that more attention be paid to constructing organization-wide standards and small group norms that encourage and reward dialogue and learning from errors. In virtual environments or in fluid groups (groups with frequent changes in membership), intraprofessional and interpersonal conflict avoidance is the norm; the ensuing misunderstandings and mistrust tend to limit collaborative or cooperative behavior and ultimately affect team performance and patient outcomes. The acceptance of professional differences and the proactive examination of errors help to create opportunities for inclusive communication, understanding, and trust, and pave the way for collaborative endeavors between disciplines and shared ownership of team outcomes (Doucet et al., 2001; Ratcheva, 2009; Sampath et al., 2021).

Sustainable collaborative environments for interprofessional healthcare teams require a collectively constructed core of prescriptive (dos) and proscriptive (don'ts) group norms or ground rules that encourage interaction at intrapersonal, interpersonal, and systems levels (Nash, 2008; National Academies, 2019; Tannenbaum et al., 2021; Pype et al., 2018; Mertens et al., 2019; Bedwell et al., 2012; Trzeciak & Mazzarelli, 2019). The Mayo Clinic's consistent adherence to norms that highlight patient-centered care and the value of teamwork has helped it retain its reputation as the most preferred provider of health care in the United States since the nineteenth century. At the Mayo Clinic, the contributions of receptionists, information managers, housekeeping personnel, therapists, nurses, physicians, pharmacists, food service, and transportation workers are all valued as an integral parts of the patient experience (Seltman & Berry, 2013). Reinforcing the norm of the centrality of patient-centered care will help team members understand that the norms and group goals take priority over personal goals and wishes.

Goals

Group goals, like norms, are both explicit and implicit. Implicit goals address the developmental processes inherent to group maturation. Focusing on, defining, and committing to the explicit work-related goals of a group is a major key to success. Commonly held goals and the collective efficacy that the achievements of these goals engender are key contributors to group performance (Silver & Bufanio, 1996). Not surprisingly, the ease of goal attainment is related to the level of goal complexity.

In the current healthcare climate, team goals for professionals are complex and require problem-solving using multiple types of data and a convergence of multiple areas of expertise and skill sets. To add to that complexity, interdisciplinary team members bring diverse professional values, individual personal goals, and goals influenced by multiple reporting relationships. It is essential that goals are not only clear but constantly revisited.

Groups that continually communicate and become more explicit with regard to the team's goals are more successful in performance. Regardless of the complexities of the team tasks and team membership, if group members are committed to the group goals, the team can succeed. If the commitment to

---

REFLECTION: Explicit and Implicit Norms in a Group

Identify the norms or rules of your work group.
Interview members of your group and ask them to identify the rules of your group.
How does your response differ from your coworkers? How is it the same?
How does the similarity/difference of perception affect the group's functioning?

the goals is low, then there is little chance of success (Locke et al., 1988; Seltman & Berry, 2013).

Roles

The inherent diversity of individual personality styles makes team members' interaction and relationships key factors in team dynamics. Researchers have studied groups of people who have a variety of styles in order to ascertain whether a particular combination of member styles has any impact on group effectiveness, outcomes, and development. Lewin (1943) observed that behavior is a function of the person and the environment, or $B = f(P, E)$. Role assumption in groups is a consequence of both an individual's personality and the context of the complex system of group dynamics that comprise team behavior and effectiveness. Roles are not necessarily attached to any individual but are assumed in response to the group's developmental needs.

Wheelan (2005) identifies three primary roles that group members assume regardless of their personality types. Task roles are needed to facilitate a project from inception to completion. Social-emotional or maintenance roles contribute to a positive group atmosphere and foster cohesion. Organizational roles like the leader, recorder, or project manager keep the group organized. Benne and Sheats (1948) classify the functional roles of group members as task, social-emotional/maintenance, and individual. Individual roles tend to disrupt group progress and weaken cohesion. **Table 3.1** provides examples of each role.

Belbin (2010) studied teamwork and observed that people in teams tend to assume various team roles, which alternate in their dominance depending upon the developmental stage of the group's activities. The nine roles where categorized into the following three groups: Action oriented, people oriented, and thought oriented. The action-oriented group includes shaper (SH), implementer (IMP), and completer–finisher (CF) roles. The people-oriented group includes coordinator (CO), team worker (TW), and resource investigator (RI) roles. The thought-oriented group includes plant (PL), monitor–evaluator (ME), and specialist (SP) roles. Each team role is associated with typical behavioral and interpersonal strengths and weaknesses. Belbin identifies the latter as "allowable weaknesses"—areas to be aware of and potentially improve upon (**Table 3.2**).

A group that is composed of members who assume only those roles related to job completion while ignoring the roles that engage and facilitate member participation runs the risk of diminished cohesion, unmanaged conflict, and apathy. All of these negatively affect the sustainability of good performance and successful outcomes. Groups that are stymied in a quagmire

Table 3.1 Benne and Sheats's Group Member Roles

Initiator/contributor	Encourager	Aggressor
Information seeker/giver	Harmonizer	Blocker
Coordinator	Compromiser	Disrupter
Evaluator	Includer	Dominator
Energizer	Follower	
Procedural technician		

Data from Benne, K. & Sheats, P. (1948). Functional roles of group members. *Journal of Social Issues*, 4(2), 41–49.

Table 3.2 Belbin's Team Roles

Thought Oriented (TO)		
Plant	■ Creative, imaginative, unorthodox ■ Solves difficult problems	■ Ignores incidentals ■ Too preoccupied to communicate effectively
Monitor Evaluator	■ Sober, strategic, and discerning ■ Sees all positions ■ Judges accurately	■ Lacks drive and ability to inspire others
Specialist	■ Single minded, self-starting, dedicated ■ Provides knowledge and skills in rare supply	■ Contributes on only a narrow front ■ Dwells on technicalities
Action Oriented (AO)		
Shaper	■ Challenging, dynamic ■ Thrives on pressure ■ Has the drive and courage to overcome obstacles	■ Prone to provocation ■ Offends people's feelings
Implementer	■ Disciplined, reliable, conservative, and efficient ■ Turns ideas into practical actions	■ Somewhat inflexible ■ Slow to respond to new possibilities
Completer/Finisher	■ Painstaking, conscientious, anxious ■ Searches out errors and omissions ■ Polishes and perfects	■ Inclined to worry unduly ■ Reluctant to delegate
People Oriented (PO)		
Team Worker	■ Cooperative, mild, perceptive, and diplomatic ■ Listens ■ Builds, averts friction	■ Indecisive in crunch situations
Resource Investigator	■ Extrovert, enthusiastic, and communicative ■ Explores opportunities ■ Develops contacts	■ Overly optimistic ■ Loses interest once initial enthusiasm has passed
Coordinator	■ Mature, confident; a good chairperson ■ Clarifies goals, promotes decision-making ■ Delegates well	■ Can be seen as manipulative ■ Offloads personal work

of conflicting emotions or that are burdened with members who are myopically focused on their personal agenda will never get any work done. These scenarios can negatively impact healthcare teams who routinely deal with issues related to complex medical decision-making and the resultant interventions that will impact a patient's lifestyle and quality of life. Throughout the life of every group of health professionals, leaders and members must be alert enough to recognize what roles need to be assumed and to be flexible enough to assume the roles that will sustain optimum group functioning and consistently positive patient outcomes.

The attempt to carry out group roles as described is further complicated by the many other personal and professional roles that are held by members of healthcare teams. While a primary challenge for all team members is to separate personal needs and roles from the team needs and roles, healthcare professionals must also juggle team and discipline-related roles that often conflict at the intraprofessional and interprofessional levels. Perceived roles and responsibilities may diverge based on variations in professional socialization, experience, and organizational expectations. Some professionals—often from the same discipline—may see themselves as primarily responsible for the physiology of care, while others believe they need to incorporate the contextual aspects of the illness experience in their treatment planning (Doucet et al., 2001). When faced with budget restrictions in a rehabilitation department, does the physical therapist on the team focus her energy on advocating for the physical therapy equipment budget or facilitating a group discussion regarding prioritizing the needs of the department? The answer depends on how group, member, and contextual issues are negotiated. Each member of the healthcare team is faced with similar decisions about role choices. These choices will affect the culture, development, and performance of the team and ultimately determine the nature of patient outcomes (Freshman et al., 2010).

Communication Styles

In spite of the role differentiation that exists among the disciplines, holistic approaches to health care can engender role overlap, ambiguity, and boundary management challenges (Gray, 2008; Klein, 2010; Nash, 2008). Teams that leverage common ground as well as disciplinary differences through well-constructed and maintained communication strategies are likely to demonstrate sustained high performance and achieve positive patient outcomes

(Drinka & Clark, 2000; Gittell, 2009). The most successful teams, whether in face-to-face or virtual environments, are characterized by members who are sensitive to the orientation of others and communicate often and equitably (Wooley et al., 2015; Trzeciak & Mazzarelli, 2019).

The first step in productive communication is to get the attention of the person with whom one is trying to communicate. Team members who understand that communication styles often reflect learning styles and professional orientation will be most successful if they take the time to adjust their communication style to complement the styles of the people with whom they are communicating. People who are action oriented are interested and tend to talk about objectives, results, performance, and productivity. Strategies, organization, and facts tend to pique the attention of those who are process oriented. People who are idea oriented are interested in concept development and innovation, while those with a people orientation focus their communication on values, beliefs, and relationship building (Youker, 1996).

While the previous examples give an indication of *how* communication is carried out and received, the following model provides some insight into *what* is communicated. Conscious attention to *how* and *what* is communicated allows for more mindful, strategic, and effective communication in virtual and face-to-face teams.

The Johari window (Luft & Ingham, 1950) is a classic model for identifying and improving an individual's relationship with a group or a group's relationships with other groups. While the discussion that follows addresses the model from an individual perspective, the concepts are applicable to groups as individual entities within organizations, where *others* refers to other groups.

The model is represented as a square that is divided into four window panes or perspectives as shown in **Figure 3.1** and is arranged as follows:

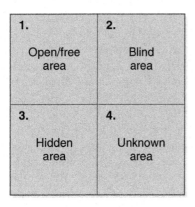

Figure 3.1 The Johari window.

Based on Luft, J., & Ingham, H. (1950). The Johari window, a graphic model of interpersonal awareness. *Proceedings of the Western Training Laboratory in group development*. University of California, Los Angeles.

Quadrant 1: Open/free area—what is known by the individual person and also known by others

Quadrant 2: Blind area—what is known by others but unknown to the individual

Quadrant 3: Hidden area—what is known by the individual and consciously hidden from others

Quadrant 4: Unknown area—what is unknown to both the individual and others

The panes/areas expand and contract to reflect the proportion of individual or group knowledge about an area. In newly formed groups, for instance, the open area is small since newly assembled groups of people know relatively little about one another. As groups mature, the open area increases as more information is shared and more cooperation and collaboration ensue. If open areas remain diminished, the group may be vulnerable to misunderstanding, mistrust, and confusion, and delay progress toward maturity. The ultimate goal for team members is to increase the size of the open area and decrease the size of the other areas through positive communication. The blind area is also known as the "bad breath area" because an individual is unaware

of something that is known by everyone else. In the case of an individual, this could be a habit such as constantly glancing at a cell phone during a meeting—unaware that the other members of the group perceive this as disrespectful. Asking for and providing constructive feedback reduces this area.

While it is appropriate to use discretion when disclosing personal or private information, feelings and information related to work proves only be helpful if they are allowed into the open area. The process of disclosure—exposing relevant information and feelings—reduces the hidden area and further expands the open area. So a group member might disclose that he/she feels disrespected when someone is checking a cell phone during a meeting or conversation. The unknown area contains information such as unconscious needs, motivations, or inherent abilities that are unrecognized by the individual or the group (**Figure 3.2**). By examining the unknown area, individuals begin to understand that perceptions of present situations may be rooted in past experiences and that the insecurity or anger that may have been experienced during a difficult childhood may be a hot button that is easily triggered by a difficult interaction in the present.

With the realization that our perceptions of present situations are formed through the lens of our own life experiences, we begin to seek information from others in order to construct a more complete picture. The ability to separate our perceptions from actuality allows us to become emotionally independent, no longer bound by automatic negative responses to triggers or hot buttons, and better able to make strategic choices regarding our actions and reactions.

If the unknown area is not reduced, the group runs the risk of not realizing individual talents and remains bound by old ways of knowing and reacting. The chances of self-actualization and motivation to become engaged in the group's work is diminished.

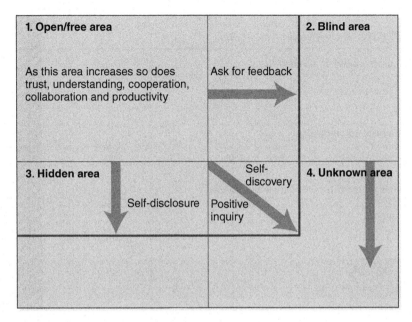

Figure 3.2 Feedback, self-disclosure, and the Johari window.

Data from Luft, J., & Ingham, H. (1950). The Johari window, a graphic model of interpersonal awareness. *Proceedings of the Western Training Laboratory in group development.* University of California, Los Angeles.

This type of awareness can be sparked through self-discovery, observations by others, and methods of inquiry that encourage mutual discovery. Communication is not always about positive experiences. Sometimes confrontation is necessary. Using positive confrontation strategies as described in the reflection can be productive (Stone Foundation, n.d.).

Leaders and members who use positive communication to facilitate self-discovery, solicit and provide constructive feedback, and foster the free flow of information create a psychologically safe environment that engenders creativity, productivity, and sustained high performance (Trzeciak & Mazzarelli, 2019; Tannenbaum et al., 2021; Mertins et al., 2019; Dinh et al., 2020).

REFLECTION: A positive confrontation

One month ago, the institution implemented a new scheduling system that resulted in a four-day workweek. A staff member has been coming in late and missing 25 percent of his treatment sessions. You are meeting with the staff member to discuss lateness.

Start the conversation with a positive statement.
I care about you, and there is a problem that I would like to work with you to solve.
State how you feel rather than being accusatory
I feel very concerned when treatment sessions are routinely missed.
Be flexible. Allow for the possibility that you may not be right
Help me to understand the situation from your point of view.
Respond to defensive deflection...but stay on focus
I understand you car pool with someone from the billing office, but for right now I would like us to stay focused on lateness and the impact on patient care.

(continues)

REFLECTION: A positive confrontation   (continued)

Reinforce commonality of purpose
I know that we agree that quality patient care is our most important focus.

Acknowledge your part in the problem
Maybe I did not make it clear that the 4-day workweek would necessitate scheduling clients one hour earlier.

Make the desired outcome clear
I understand that you may need to make alternative commuting plans. Between now and Monday, I will not schedule your patients during the first hour. By Monday, I expect that you will be ready to treat patients at 7:30 a.m.

Set boundaries if the interaction does not go well
Let me be clear. The 4-day workweek is now official institutional policy. Staff can no longer negotiate for alternative work hours.

CASE STUDY   Communication Style Match

Members of the interprofessional team on a geriatric unit (physician, nurse, physical therapist, occupational therapist, and social worker) are meeting to discuss patient safety on the unit. During the previous quarter, falls increased by 10 percent. Analysis of the incident reports indicates that an examination of the fall prevention program that is offered jointly by nursing, physical therapy, and occupational therapy is indicated. The team is meeting with the goal of designing a revised fall prevention program for the unit. The proposed program will need to be based in the most current evidence, ensure the safety of the patients, and be cost effective. All four styles of communication noted previously in this chapter—action oriented (physician and physical therapist), process oriented (occupational therapist), people oriented (social worker), and idea oriented (nurse)—are represented. The leader (in this case, it is the physical therapist) is an identified action-oriented communicator. In preparation for the first meeting, she reviews strategies for adjusting her communication style to the team members and prepares her opening remarks. Her remarks might vary depending on how she perceives the other members of the group. She lists pointers for addressing the others based on their communication styles, along with alternate statements for each type.

Communicating with an Action-Oriented Person

- Focus on the results first.
- State your best recommendation.
- Emphasize the practicality of your idea.

At the first meeting, if the other members are action oriented, the physical therapist might say, "The purpose of this group is to address the increased number of falls on the unit this last quarter. We need to revise the fall prevention program that is currently offered. I recommend that we construct a program around the three components that have been identified in the literature. Developing a fall prevention program that includes exercise, fall prevention, and environmental components is the most effective focus."

Communicating with a Process-Oriented Person

- State the facts.
- Present your thoughts in a logical manner.
- Include options with pros and cons.
- Do not rush the person.

If the other members are process oriented, the physical therapist might say, "The purpose of this group is to address the increased number of falls on the unit this last quarter. We need to revise the fall prevention program that is currently offered. One option that we may choose to pursue is to do a literature review on the efficacy of fall prevention and develop a custom program for our unit. We may also explore the option of purchasing existing modules. What are your thoughts?"

Communicating with a People-Oriented Person

- Allow for small talk at the beginning of a session.
- Stress the relationship between the proposal and the people concerned.
- Show how the idea worked well in the past.
- Show respect for people.

The physical therapist might say to such a group, "The purpose of this group is to address the increased number of falls on the unit this last quarter. Each of you has been chosen for this team because of your demonstrated commitment to patient safety. You are the experts in the day-to-day care of our patients. One area that we may need to consider is a revision of the fall prevention program that we currently offer. Institutions that are similar to ours have reported great success in reducing patient falls using a combination of exercise, addressing fear of falling, and modifying the environment."

Communicating with an Idea-Oriented Person

- Allow enough time for discussion.
- Do not get impatient when they go off on tangents.
- Be broad and conceptual in your opening.

The physical therapist could address this type of group by saying, "As key staff members on this geriatric unit, you have demonstrated your commitment to patient safety. I have asked each of you to be a member of this team because we have yet another safety concern. The purpose of this group is to address the increased number of falls on the unit this last quarter. We need to revise the fall prevention program that is currently offered. Yes, the plan for tornado drills has been effective. Is there anything that we learned during the development and implementation of the tornado drill policy that we can bring to the creation of a fall prevention program?"

By acknowledging the presence of a variety of communication styles and adjusting her approach, this leader has demonstrated respect for team members and hopefully avoided potential problems in team communication at the beginning of this important project.

Communication Networks

In the 1950s, Leavitt (1951) graphically described common communication networks in small groups using circles and arrows to illustrate how information is processed and distributed. Simple tasks that require the processing of limited amounts of information are most efficiently carried out in centralized networks like the wheel, where one person serves as the hub for information exchange (**Figure 3.3A**). More complex tasks, which require the processing of large amounts of complex information, are most efficiently handled by decentralized networks of communication such as a circle, where there is a free-flowing information exchange among all

participants (**Figure 3.3B**). In the current healthcare environment, a spider web might be a more appropriate metaphor for the complex communication networks through which vast amounts of complex information travels with the help of information and communication technologies (Mo, 2016).

Attention to the analysis of social networks and information exchange is crucial to understanding the problem-solving and intraorganizational learning capacity of complex health systems. Knowledge-intensive healthcare organizations depend upon high-functioning teams with communication networks that emphasize a free flow of information that is unconstrained by hierarchy or discipline (Stokols et al., 2008; Gray, 2008; Agneessens & Wittek, 2012).

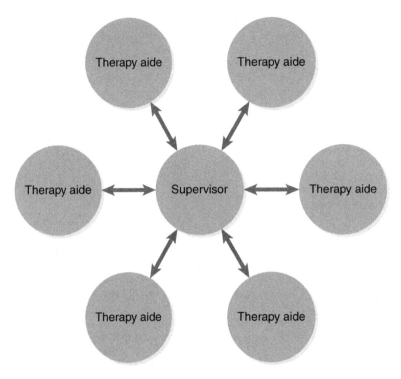

Figure 3.3A A centralized network.

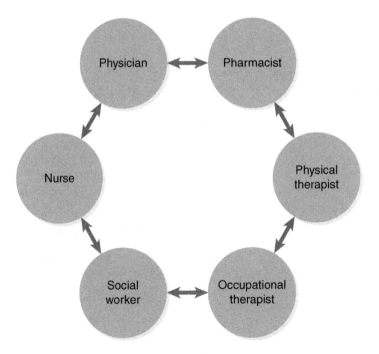

Figure 3.3B A decentralized network.

Systematic observation of communication patterns provides insight into how the flow of information is related to power and influence within teams. Lower-status individuals are less likely to express their thoughts and feelings in groups with people of higher status. Higher-status individuals tend to do more of the talking. According to the Institute of Medicine (2003), hierarchical communication patterns are partially responsible for medical errors. Additional challenges to communication may also exist along gender and generational lines (Spector, 2010). Communication patterns in teams that employ collaborative processes like directness, mutual understanding, and full participation of members tends to create a climate of psychological safety across the hierarchies and results in more inclusive communication and more effective and efficient exchange of information (Meads & Ashcroft, 2005; Nembhard & Edmondson, 2006; Edmondson, 2019).

Healthcare organizations are composed of a diverse network of health professionals, patients, and caregivers who must leverage each other's expertise by coordinating the exchange and flow of highly complex data. Health information technology (HIT) professionals can help to design information exchange strategies that distribute leadership and facilitate accountability and engagement of every member of the team (Gray, 2008; Hammick et al., 2009;

Christopherson et al., 2015). HIT can support collaborative practice when its design is informed by the culture, values, and goals of the health system. Health professionals' contributions to the electronic health record usually address patient's history, plan of care, assessments, education, and transitions or "handoffs" to other levels of care. Each of these areas provides opportunities for interprofessional communication, role delineation and overlap, collaboration, and shared decision-making. If a health system's goal is to provide evidence-based, interprofessional, patient-centered care, HIT tools must be designed to support those goals. The electronic health record, enhanced with contextually relevant hardware and software, can become a nexus for various viewpoints that informs collaborative, patient-centered decision-making (Christopherson et al., 2015). High-quality feedback among interdependent team members yields high levels of cohesion, satisfaction, and performance in teams (Garman, 2010; Gittell, 2009; Goleman et al., 2002).

Online communities and social media platforms offer opportunities for healthcare providers and healthcare consumers to collaborate and share practical knowledge in spite of geographical distance, scheduling conflicts, and status differentials. While it is true that this type of increased interaction can facilitate empathy, trust, and cohesion, technology alone does not create collaborative cultures.

COMMUNICATION NETWORKS

Simple tasks, like stocking supply closets in the therapy gyms, requires processing limited amounts of information and can be most efficiently carried out in a centralized network like the wheel. A supervisor (hub of the wheel) might direct therapy aides via email or face-to-face communication. More complex tasks, like developing a comprehensive patient discharge plan, requires processing large amounts of complex information and might be most efficiently handled by decentralized networks of communication among the physician, nurse, therapists, social worker, and other professionals, using face-to-face and virtual conferencing with the electronic health record.

A culture of collaboration is an important prerequisite for sustainable integration of technology and health care (Norman & Yip, 2013; Christopherson et al., 2015; Kotlarsky et al., 2015). Institutions that invest in the development of relationships through formal structures that support frequent and consistent time allocation for team meetings—face-to-face and virtual—will find that gains in patient outcomes will mirror gains in social capital (Drinka & Clark, 2000; Ghaye, 2005; Gittell, 2009; Institute of Medicine, 2003; Lawrence, 2002; Ratcheva, 2009; Norman & Yip, 2013).

Administrators and clinicians find it difficult to justify taking time away from direct patient care in order to attend meetings because the fast-paced healthcare environment places time at a premium. However, recent healthcare reforms have linked reimbursement to patient outcomes such as length of stay, readmission rates, and patient satisfaction rather than the number of procedures and services provided. While one could argue that the time spent in meetings is not reimbursable, it would be hard to deny that the improvements in team communication and performance positively affect team sustainability and patient outcomes.

Collaborative, participative environments engender increased knowledge and mutual respect among health team members. Increased awareness of the expertise available to the team will facilitate the team's ability to distribute leadership based on the nature of the challenge, and disciplinary boundaries can become points of connection and innovation rather than points of contention (Drinka & Clark, 2000; Gray, 2008; Meads & Ashcroft, 2005; Wheatley, 2006). Leaders who are willing to trust in the diverse wisdom and singular intent of the collective actively encourage and seek participation from all members of the team. Consequently, communication disparities are mitigated and psychologically safe team environments are created. All members are encouraged to contribute, exercise leadership, and be personally engaged and accountable for the team outcomes (Nembhard & Edmondson, 2006; Wheatley, 2006).

CASE STORY Technology and Communication in an Interprofessional Setting

At Austill's Rehabilitation Services, Inc., all managers were able to use a secure network that allowed 24:7 access to email, voicemail, and a custom-designed database, which provided client information. Four hundred school-based occupational, physical, and speech therapists had access to secure accountability, billing, and data collection systems. WEB-based IEPs (individualized educational plans) expanded interprofessional team communication. Each team member's student assessment, summary, recommendations, and daily progress were communicated to the team, which facilitated consistent collaboration even though therapists were geographically distant.

We used Skype, FaceTime, and videoconferencing to interview potential employees, supervise staff, participate in university-based educational activities, and have access to specialists who provided real-time support to the therapists. Technology has helped facilitate interprofessional communication and skill development within the organization and with partners outside of the organization, and has positively impacted client outcomes.

—Rebecca Austill-Clausen, MS, OTR/L, FAOTA, Founder, Austill's Rehabilitation Services, Inc. Currently, Reiki Master, President of Complementary Health Works, Inc., Downingtown, PA

REFLECTION: Identifying Opportunities for Collaboration

Health professionals' contributions to the electronic health records usually address the following areas. In your setting, which areas provide opportunities for communication, collaboration, role delineation, role overlap, and shared decision-making?

History
Plan of care
Assessments
Education
Transitions (hand offs)

References

Agneessens, F., & Wittek, R. (2012). Where do intra-organizational advice relations come from? The role of informal status and social capital in social exchange. *Social Networks, 34*(3), 333–345.

Bedwell, W., Ramsay, S., & Salas, E. (2012). Helping fluid teams work: A research agenda for effective team adaptation in healthcare. *Translational Behavioral Medicine, 2,* 504–509 doi: 10.1007/s13142-012-0177-9

Belbin, R. (2010). *Team roles at work* (2nd ed.). Butterworth Heinemann/Elsevier.

Benne, K., & Sheats, P. (1948). Functional roles of group members. *Journal of Social Issues, 4*(2), 41–49.

Christopherson, T., Troseth, M., & Clingerman, E. (2015). Informatics-enabled interprofessional education and collaborative practice: A framework-driven approach. *Journal of Interprofessional Education & Practice, 1,* 10–15.

Dinh, J., Traylor, A., Kilcullen, M., Perez, J., Schweissing, E., Venkatesh, A., & Salas, E. (2020). Cross-disciplinary care: A systematic review on teamwork processes in health care. *Small Group Research, 51*(1), 125–166. doi: 10.1177/1046496419872002

Doucet, H., Larouche, J., & Melchin, K. (2001). *Ethical deliberation in multiprofessional health care teams.* University of Ottawa Press.

Drinka, T., & Clark, P. (2000). *Health care teamwork: Interdisciplinary practice and teaching.* Auburn House.

Edmondson, A. (2019). *The fearless organization: Creating psychological safety in the workplace for learning, innovation and growth.* John Wiley & Sons.

Freshman, B., Rubino, L., & Chassiakos, Y. (2010). *Collaboration across the disciplines in health care.* Jones and Bartlett Publishers.

Garman, A. (2010). Leadership development in the interdisciplinary context. In B. Freshman, L. Rubino, & Y. Chassiakos (Eds.), *Collaboration across the disciplines in health care* (pp. 43–64). Jones and Bartlett Publishers.

Ghaye, T. (2005). *Developing the reflective healthcare team.* Blackwell Publishing, Ltd.

Gittell, J. (2009). *High performance healthcare: Using the power of relationships to achieve quality, efficiency and resilience.* McGraw-Hill.

Goleman, D., Boyatzis, R., & McKee, A. (2002). *Primal leadership: Learning to lead with emotional intelligence.* Harvard Business School Press.

Gray, B. (2008). Enhancing transdisciplinary research through collaborative leadership. *American Journal of Preventive Medicine, 35*(2S), s124–s132.

Hammick, M., Freeth, D. S., Copperman, J., & Goodsman, D. (2009). *Being interprofessional.* Polity Press.

Institute of Medicine, Committee on the Health Professions Education Summit; Greiner, A. C., & Knebel, E. (Eds.). (2003). *Health professions education: A bridge to quality.* National Academies Press.

Klein, J. (2010). *Creating interdisciplinary campus cultures: A model for strength and sustainability.* Jossey-Bass.

Kotlarsky, J., van den Hooff, B., & Houtman, L. (2015). Are we on the same page? Knowledge boundaries and transactive memory system development in cross functional teams. *Communication Research, 42*(3), 319–344.

Lawrence, D. (2002). *From chaos to care: The promise of team based medicine.* Perseus Publishing.

Leavitt, H. (1951). Some effects of certain communication patterns on group performance. *Journal of Abnormal and Social Psychology, 46,* 38–50.

Lewin, K. (1943). Defining the "field at a given time." *Psychological Review, 50,* 292–310.

Locke, E. A., Latham, G. P., & Erez, M. (1988). The determinants of goal commitment. *Academy of Management Review, 1,* 23–39.

Luft, J., & Ingham, H. (1950). The Johari window, a graphic model of interpersonal awareness. *Proceedings of the Western Training Laboratory in group development.* University of California Los Angeles.

Meads, G., & Ashcroft, J. (2005). *The case for interprofessional collaboration in health and social care.* Blackwell Publishing.

Mertens, F., de Gendt, A., Deveugele, M., van Hecke, A., & Pype, P. (2019). Interprofessional collaboration within fluid teams: Community nurses' experiences with palliative home care. *Journal of Clinical Nursing, 28,* 3680–3690. https://doi.org/10.1111/jocn.1496

Mo, G. (2016). Examining cross-disciplinary communication's impact on multidisciplinary collaborations: Implications for innovations. *Information, Communication & Society,* DOI: 10.1080/1369118X.2016.1139611

Nash, J. (2008). Transdisciplinary training: Key components and prerequisites for success. *American Journal of Preventative Medicine, 35*(2S), s133–s140.

National Academies of Sciences, Engineering, and Medicine. (2019). *Taking action against clinician burnout: A systems approach to professional well-being.* The National Academies Press. https://doi.org/10.17226/25521

Nembhard, I., & Edmondson, A. (2006). Making it safe: The effects of leader inclusiveness and professional status on psychological safety and improvement efforts in health care teams. *Journal of Organizational Behavior, 27,* 941–966.

Norman, C., & Yip, A. (2013). Chapter 34: Designing for health promotion, social innovation, and complexity: the CoNEKTR Model for wicked problems. In J. Sturmberg & C. Martin (Eds.), *Handbook of systems and complexity in health* (pp. 581–593). Springer Science+Business Media.

O'Daniel, M., & Rosenstein, A. H. (2008). Chapter 33: Professional communication and team collaboration. In R. G. Hughes (Ed.), *Patient safety and quality: An evidence-based handbook for nurses* (pp. 271–284). Agency for Healthcare Research and Quality. http://www.ncbi.nlm.nih.gov/books/NBK2637/

Pype, P., Mertens, F., Helewaut, F., & Krystallidou, D. (2018). Healthcare teams as complex adaptive systems: Understanding team behaviour through team members' perception of interpersonal interaction. *BMC Health Services Research, 18,* 570. https://doi.org/10.1186/s12913-018-3392-3

Ratcheva, V. (2009). Integrating diverse knowledge through boundary spanning processes: The case for multidisciplinary project teams. *International Journal of Project Management, 27,* 206–215.

Sampath, B., Rakover, J., Baldoza, K., Mate, K., Lenoci-Edwards, J., & Barker, P. (2021). *Whole system quality: A unified approach to building responsive, resilient health care systems* (IHI White Paper). Institute for Healthcare Improvement. www.ihi.orgief.com

Seltman, K., & Berry, L. (2013). Mayo Clinic: Making complex healthcare simpler. In J. Sturmberg & C. Martin (Eds.), *Handbook of systems and complexity in health* (pp. 685–696). Springer Science + Business Media.

Sherif, M. (1936). *The psychology of social norms.* Harper & Row.

Silver, W., & Bufanio, K. (1996). The impact of group efficacy and group goals on group task performance. *Small Group Research, 27,* 347–359.

Spector, N. (2010). Interprofessional collaboration: A nursing perspective. In F. Freshman, L. Rubino, & Y. Chassiakos (Eds.), *Collaboration across the disciplines in healthcare* (p. 107). Jones and Bartlett Publishers.

Stokols, D., Hall, K., Tylor, B., & Moser, R. (2008). The science of team science. *American Journal of Preventative Medicine, 35*(2S), s77–s89.

Stone Foundation Counseling Group. (n.d.). *The art of healthy confrontation: 8 steps.* http://thestonefoundation.com

Tannenbaum, S., Traylor, A., Thomas, E., & Salas, E. (2021). Managing teamwork in the face of pandemic: Evidence-based tips. *BMJ Quality and Safety, 30,* 59–63.

Torrens, P. (2010). The health care team members: Who are they and what do they do? In B. Freshman, L. Rubino, & Y. Chassiakos (Eds.), *Collaboration across the disciplines in health care* (pp. 1–19). Jones and Bartlett Publishers.

Trzeciak, S., & Mazzarrelli, A. (2019). *Compassionomics: The revolutionary scientific evidence that caring makes a difference.* Studer Group.

Wheatley, M. (2006). *Leadership and the new science: Discovering order in a chaotic world* (3rd ed.). Berrett-Koehler Publishers, Inc.

Wheelan, S. (2005). *Group process: A developmental perspective* (2nd ed.). Allyn & Bacon.

Wooley, A., Malone, T., & Chabris, C. (2015, January 16). Why some teams are smarter than others. *New York Times.* http://www.nytimes.com

Youker, R. (1996). Communication style instrument: A team building tool. In *PMI seminars & symposium proceedings* (pp. 796–799). Project Management Institute.

Team and Group Development Activities

Activity 1: How Much of a Team Is Your Group?

In Chapter 1, the difference between a group and a team is described on a continuum. At one end of the spectrum, a group refers to any group of people with something in common and at the other end, a team refers to people who must work together to reach a common goal or outcome. Identify three groups or teams that of which you have been a part. Place them on a continuum and provide a rationale for your decision.

Activity 2: *I* and *We*

From your experience as a member or leader in an interprofessional team, develop two cases to analyze from the "I" and the "We" perspective. Specifically, identify the following times:

- You made a decision in the team's interest and not your interest. What was the effect on you? On the members of the team?
- You made a decision in the patient's interest and not your interest. What was the effect on you? On the patient?

Activity 3: TOPS: Team Orientation and Performance Survey

TOPS is a survey that can help you determine where the energy of the group is focused. When you fill this out, remember that this is your perception of the team. Other team members may see it differently. Rank the endings of each sentence according to how well each ending describes your team. Enter a 4 for the sentence ending that *best* describes your team now, down to a 1 for the sentence ending that seems *least* like your team. Be sure to rank all the endings for each sentence unit.

Utilizing the scores on the TOPS, refer to the text for a description of the developmental level that is most like your team. At which group developmental stage is your team? Is the TOPS score consistent with your experience of the team? What strategies could you use as a team member or leader to positively impact the team's development?

1. Team members	___ talk about topics that are safe.	___ argue with each other.	___ are open with the group about their thoughts and feelings.	___ talk openly about issues and concerns and give constructive feedback.
2. Team members	___ tend to agree.	___ disagree with each other.	___ offer relevant facts, opinions, and ideas during group discussions.	___ resolve conflicts before moving on to other subjects.
3. Team members	___ don't voice differences of opinion.	___ don't handle conflicts constructively.	___ can be candid about differences of opinion.	___ listen to different points of view and use the differences to create more effective outcomes.
4. Team members	___ depend on the leader for direction.	___ depend on the leader for direction yet resent the direction the leader gives.	___ utilize the leader as an advisor, and the leader delegates responsibility for process, decisions, and implementation to the team.	___ share the leadership function.
5. Team members	___ direct almost all comments toward the leader.	___ vary in their support of the leader.	___ have a positive evaluation of the leader's abilities.	___ recognize and utilize the leader for his or her strengths.
6. Team members	___ do not disagree with the leader.	___ tend to disagree with the leader.	___ trust that the leader is giving them the information and authority they need to get the job done.	___ see the leader as a resource to help them get the job done.
7. Team members	___ have a purpose and goals that are unclear.	___ disagree about goals.	___ agree about the team goals.	___ have goals that are well defined and measurable.
8. Team members	___ have roles that are unclear.	___ are confused about roles, tasks, and responsibilities.	___ have role assignments that are defined and match their abilities.	___ understand each other's roles, and they are not overly rigid.
9. The team	___ has a structure and processes that are organized by the leader.	___ feels disorganized.	___ is talking about and agreeing on how to organize work.	___ is well organized and can adjust processes and procedures to fit the work task.

10. Team members	___ are concerned with being liked.	___ want recognition for the unique skills and abilities they bring to the team.	___ behave with trust, respect, and care toward one another and what they bring to the team.	___ have a *we* orientation rather than a *me* orientation.
11. Team members	___ do not feel like a team.	___ have expressed frustration within the group.	___ communicate appreciation for each other's talents and capabilities.	___ are safe taking interpersonal risk.
12. Team members	___ are concerned with fitting in.	___ feel tension in the group.	___ trust each other's intentions.	___ can implement decisions that are best for the team as a whole even if they conflict with individual preferences.
Totals	DI =	CC =	TS =	WP =

DI = dependency and inclusion; CC = counterdependency and conflict; TS = trust and structure; WP = energy in work and productivity.
Developed by Felice Tilin for GroupWorks Consulting, LLC (owned by Felice Tilin) 2009 Felice Tilin. All rights reserved.

Activity 4: Team Goal Setting

The most effective team goals are specific, measurable, attainable, relevant, and time bound (SMART). The following questions will help you and your team to create SMART goals. Think of a short-term project that is important for your team to accomplish. Use these questions to inform your goal development and evaluate whether your goals have been achieved.

- What goals does the organization expect this team to achieve?
- Can we operationally define the goal(s)?
- Are the goals clear to each member of the team?
- Does it tell the team who, what, when, where, which, and why?
  - *What:* What do we want to accomplish?
  - *Why:* Specific reasons, purpose, or benefits of accomplishing the goal.
  - *Who:* Who is involved?

- *Where and when:* Identify locations and time lines.
- *Which:* Identify requirements and constraints.

Measurable

What are the criteria for measuring progress toward the attainment of the goal? Measuring keeps a team on track, helps the team reach its target dates, and tests whether it has completed tasks, milestones, and final accomplishments.

A measurable goal will usually answer questions such as:

- How much?
- How many?
- When?

Attainable

Are the goals realistic and attainable? Does the team have the right members on it to do the job (or can it recruit these members)? Does the team have resources and the proper amount of authority? Who are the champions in the organization? How will the team get help when it needs it?

An attainable goal will usually answer the question:

- *How:* How can the goal be accomplished?

Relevant

- Who is this important to? Goals that are relevant to the superiors, the team, or the organization should receive that needed support.
- How is it relevant to each individual on the team?
- How does it support or align with other organizational goals?
- How does it align with an overall organizational strategy, organizational values, and/or its mission?

A relevant goal can answer yes to these questions:

- Is it worthwhile?
- Is this the right time?

- Does this match our other efforts/needs?
- Are we the right people to get this job done?

Time Bound

What is the target for completion? When will the team complete tasks, mini goals, and milestones? This part of the SMART goal criteria is intended to prevent goals from being overtaken by the day-to-day crises that invariably arise in an organization. A time-bound goal is intended to establish a sense of urgency.

A time-bound goal will usually answer the following questions:

- When?
- What can we do in 10 days, 10 weeks, or 10 months?
- What do we need to accomplish today?

© oxygen/Moment/Getty Images

Relationship-Centered Leadership

"If your actions inspire others to dream more, do more and become more . . . you are a leader."

— John Quincy Adams

CHAPTER 4

Perspectives on Leadership

LEARNING OBJECTIVES

1. Analyze various theories of leadership.
2. Explore the relationship of personality and leadership styles.
3. Determine how leadership is affected by the context and situation in which it is exercised.
4. Examine the relationship of emotional intelligence and leadership.
5. Investigate the competencies required for health professions leadership.
6. Identify personal leadership characteristics.

Leadership emerges as a compilation of mysteries that have been investigated for centuries. Researchers have attempted to answer questions such as: Are leaders born? Can leaders be developed? Does the environment create the leader? Is leadership emergence synonymous with leader effectiveness? What role does social dynamics have in the leadership equation? Can leadership be shared (Avolio, 2007; Zaccaro, 2007)? How and why should group members assume a leadership stance (Stoffel, 2014)? The latter questions resonate when contemplating the development and sustainability of effective interprofessional healthcare teams. An examination of the broader phenomenon of leadership provides a context for that inquiry.

Perspectives on Leadership

Leadership connotes position as well as action. Positional leadership refers to responsibility given to an individual or group of individuals to guide, direct, or control. People who are hired as managers can be considered positional leaders. However, not everyone who is a manager exercises leadership. Conversely, anyone can exercise leadership. The act of leadership or ability to lead refers to the effective use of influence and a complex dynamic that has inspired much of the research on leadership. Leadership can be simply defined as the exercise of power and influence with others. Some theorists have posited that leaders are born, while others focus on the role that social, cultural, political, and environmental factors have on the emergence of leaders.

Many perspectives regarding leadership offer intriguing views of the leadership concept, but no definitive conceptualization exists. A comprehensive review of these views is beyond the scope of this book. For the purposes of our discussion, we will focus on three broad theoretical approaches that are supported by modern-day research and are most applicable to healthcare leadership development. These approaches include personality/trait, contingency/situational, and relational theories. We will provide a summary of each of these theoretical approaches, highlight the most relevant theoretical concepts, and provide opportunities for the practical application of these concepts.

Personality and Trait Theories

Early conceptualizations of leadership focused on the "great man" theory, which hypothesized that leaders were born with certain characteristics that predisposed them to take command and lead others (Carlyle, 1841). The Zeitgeist theory credited the convergence of social, political, and individual factors with the emergence of a leader—the right person for the right time in history (Tolstoy, 1867/2010). Subsequent trait theorists, informed by the big five theory of personality described a constellation of traits that were indicative of a leadership personality.

The Big Five

The Big Five or OCEAN model of personality is a long-standing and widely accepted model that describes five personality trait continuums: **Openness** (imaginative, creative, open minded), **Conscientiousness** (goal oriented), **Extroversion** (positive attitude, sociable), **Agreeableness** (accommodating, adaptable), and **Neuroticism** (need for stability, pessimistic). Each of these traits is represented as a continuum that ranges between two extremes (e.g., introversion and extroversion) (McCrae & Costa, 1987). Over the years, researchers have continued to expand upon this model and to develop tools such as the HEXACO Personality Inventory and the Hogan Personality Inventory (HPI) to further identify the nuances of personality (Ashton et al., 2014; Hogan & Smither, R. 2008). The HEXACO includes a sixth dimension, **Honesty/Humility** (honest, sincere, fair, and modest), and uses the term "Emotionality" to describe the "Neuroticism" continuum (**Tables 4.1** and **4.2**). The HPI, on the other hand, is composed of seven primary scales: Adjustment, Ambition, Sociability, Interpersonal Sensitivity, Prudence, Inquisitiveness, and Learning Approach, which describe personal tendencies as well as social intelligence (Hogan & Hogan, 2007).

It is accepted that personality is a complex phenomenon with wide variation among individuals. However, according to this model, the "ideal leader" is resilient (low on emotionality), energetic and outgoing (high on extroversion), visionary (high on openness), competitive (low on agreeableness), and dedicated to a goal (high on conscientiousness).

Myers-Briggs Type Indicator (MBTI)

Katharine Cook Briggs and Isabel Briggs Myers based the MBTI on the hypothesis that people are born with innate personality traits (Jung, 1910/1991). The Myers-Briggs type indicator is a popular self-report survey instrument that is often used to identify preferred behavioral styles across the four dichotomies

Table 4.1 HEXACO Personality Inventory

Domain Level Scales	Facet Level Scales
Honesty-Humility	sincerity, greed avoidance, fairness, modesty
Emotionality	anxiety, dependence, sentimentality, fearfulness
Extroversion	sociability, social boldness, social self-esteem, liveliness
Agreeableness	flexibility, gentleness, forgiveness, patience
Conscientiousness	diligence, organization, perfection, prudence
Openness to new experiences	inquisitiveness, aesthetic appreciation, unconventionality, creativity

Table 4.2 Reflection: HEXACO Scale Descriptions

Which traits are most closely aligned with your characteristic behaviors?
Which traits enhance your ability to lead and which traits hinder your ability to lead?
High Low ➤

Honesty-Humility

Avoids manipulating others for personal gain	Will flatter others for personal gain
Rarely tempted to break rules	Will break rules for personal profit
Uninterested in wealth	Motivated by material gain
Does not feel entitled	Strong sense of self-importance

Emotionality

Fears physical danger	Not deterred by prospect of physical harm
Feels anxious in response to stress	Does not worry
Needs emotional support from others	Has little need to share with others
Feels empathy and attachment to others	Emotionally detached from others

eXtraversion

Positive self-image	Feels unpopular
Confident leading groups	Awkward in front of groups
Enjoys social interaction	Indifferent to social activities
Enthusiastic and energetic	Less optimistic

Agreeableness

Forgives wrongs	Holds grudges
Not judgmental	Judgmental

(continues)

Table 4.2 Reflection: HEXACO Scale Descriptions *(continued)*

Willing to compromise and cooperate	Stubborn
Even tempered	Easily angered
Conscientiousness	
Organized	Unorganized
Disciplined	Not persistent in the pursuit of goals
Accurate	Tolerant of errors
Deliberative	Impulsive
Openness to Experience	
Moved by beauty in art and nature	Unimpressed by art
Inquisitive	Not intellectually curious
Imaginative	Not creative
Interested in unusual people and ideas	Conventional

Data from: https://hexaco.org/

(extroversion/introversion, sensing/intuition, thinking/feeling, and judging/perceiving) and to provide insight into how individuals find energy, gather information, make decisions, and orient to the environment (Myers et al., 1998). While it does not identify talents, quantify intelligence, or predict leadership success, it facilitates self-awareness, which does correlate with leadership success (Goleman & Boyatzis, 2008).

Myers-Briggs Type Dichotomies

This diagram summarizes the four types of dichotomies and their related preferences based on Myers and Briggs's conceptualization.

Extroversion: *I gain energy from working with others.*	←——————→	Introversion: *I gain energy from working alone.*
Senser: *I take information from the here and now.*	←——————→	Intuiter: *I integrate information from past, present, and future.*
Thinker: *I make decisions based on logic.*	←——————→	Feeler: *I make decisions based on belief.*
Judger: *I like structure.*	←——————→	Perceiver: *I like to improvise.*

Data from Myers, I. B., McCaulley, M. H., Quenk, N. L., & Hammer, A. L. (1998). *MBTI manual: A guide to the development and use of the Myers-Briggs type indicator* (3rd ed.). Consulting Psychologists Press.

REFLECTION: MBTI Detailed Descriptions

Read the following descriptions to determine your personality and preferred behavioral style on each of the four MBTI dichotomies.

Extroversion/Introversion—How a Person Finds Energy

Extroverts (E) are energized by the outside world (people and things).	Introverts (I) are energized by being alone with their internal thoughts.
■ Draw energy from action ■ Tend to act first, then reflect, and then act again ■ Energy level tends to drop when not engaged in an activity ■ Are influenced by the expectations and attention of others ■ Enjoy working in groups	■ Draw energy from reflection ■ Prefer to reflect before acting ■ Energy tends to drop with too much external interaction ■ May defend against external demands and intrusions ■ Enjoy working alone or with a few others

Sensing/Intuiting—How a Person Takes in Information

Sensors (S) prefer to take in information in the here and now and in a precise manner.	Intuitives (N) like to take in information in a holistic and extemporaneous manner.
■ Focus on objective facts and circumstances as perceived by the senses (seeing, feeling, hearing) first ■ Have excellent powers of observation ■ Deal with how things are rather than on how they could be ■ See problems as needing specific solutions based on past information ■ Value realism	■ Focus on the big picture and underlying pattern, beyond the reach of the senses first ■ Have vivid powers of imagination ■ Focus more on how things could be rather than how they are ■ See problems as opportunities to innovate based on inspiration ■ Value imagination

Thinking/Feeling—How a Person Prefers to Make a Decision

Thinkers (T) will choose objectivity and logic when making decisions.	Feelers (F) will choose what they believe in when they make a decision.
■ Seek logic and clarity ■ Question first ■ Have an interest in data ■ Know when logic is required ■ Prefer objectivity ■ Weigh pros and cons ■ Strive to be fair	■ Seek emotional clarity ■ Accept first ■ Have an interest in people ■ Know when support is required ■ Consider impact on people ■ Weigh values ■ Strive to be compassionate

Judging/Perceiving—How a Person Prefers to Live His/Her Life

Judging (J) types like to come to closure and take action.	Perceiving (P) types like to remain open and adapt to new information.
■ Prefer matters to be settled and structured ■ Finish before deadline	■ Prefer things to be flexible and open ■ Finish task at the deadline

(continues)

REFLECTION: MBTI Detailed Descriptions   *(continued)*

■ Prefer matters to be settled and structured	■ Prefer things to be flexible and open
■ Finish before deadline	■ Finish task at the deadline
■ Like plans and goals and reducing surprises	■ Like to see what turns up and enjoy surprises
■ Quickly commit to a plan	■ Reserve the right to change a plan
■ See routines as effective	■ See routines as limiting
■ Trust the plan	■ Trust the process

REFLECTION: MBTI 16 Types at a Glance

Read the following descriptions and match your MBTI findings to interpret your personality and preferred behavioral style on each of the four MBTI dichotomies.

The 16 MBTI Types

ISTJ (Introversion, Sensing, Thinking, Judging)

Quiet, serious, earn success by thoroughness and dependability. Practical, matter-of-fact, realistic, and responsible. Decide logically what should be done and work toward it steadily, regardless of distractions. Take pleasure in making everything orderly and organized—their work, their home, their life. Value traditions and loyalty.

ISFJ (Introversion, Sensing, Feeling, Judging)

Quiet, friendly, responsible, and conscientious. Committed and steady in meeting their obligations. Thorough, painstaking, and accurate. Loyal, considerate, notice and remember specifics about people who are important to them, concerned with how others feel. Strive to create an orderly and harmonious environment at work and at home.

INFJ (Introversion, Intuition, Feeling, Judging)

Seek meaning and connection in ideas, relationships, and material possessions. Want to understand what motivates people and are insightful about others. Conscientious and committed to their firm values. Develop a clear vision about how best to serve the common good. Organized and decisive in implementing their vision.

INTJ (Introversion, Intuition, Thinking, Judging)

Have original minds and great drive for implementing their ideas and achieving their goals. Quickly see patterns in external events and develop long-range explanatory perspectives. When committed, organize a job and carry it through. Skeptical and independent, have high standards of competence and performance—for themselves and others.

ISTP (Introversion, Sensing, Thinking, Perceiving)

Tolerant and flexible, quiet observers until a problem appears, then act quickly to find workable solutions. Analyze what makes things work and readily get through large amounts of data to isolate the core of practical problems. Interested in cause and effect, organize facts using logical principles, value efficiency.

ISFP (Introversion, Sensing, Feeling, Perceiving)

Quiet, friendly, sensitive, and kind. Enjoy the present moment, what's going on around them. Like to have their own space and to work within their own time frame. Loyal and committed to their values and to people who are important to them. Dislike disagreements and conflicts; do not force their opinions or values on others.

INFP (Introversion, Intuition, Feeling, Perceiving)

Idealistic, loyal to their values and to people who are important to them. Want an external life that is congruent with their values. Curious, quick to see possibilities, can be catalysts for implementing ideas. Seek to understand people and to help them fulfill their potential. Adaptable, flexible, and accepting unless a value is threatened.

INTP (Introversion, Intuition, Thinking, Perceiving)

Seek to develop logical explanations for everything that interests them. Theoretical and abstract, interested more in ideas than in social interaction. Quiet, contained, flexible, and adaptable. Have unusual ability to focus in depth to solve problems in their area of interest. Skeptical, sometimes critical, always analytical.

ESTP (Extroversion, Sensing, Thinking, Perceiving)

Flexible and tolerant, they take a pragmatic approach focused on immediate results. Theories and conceptual explanations bore them—they want to act energetically to solve the problem. Focus on the here-and-now, spontaneous, enjoy each moment that they can be active with others. Enjoy material comforts and style. Learn best through doing.

ESFP (Extroversion, Sensing, Feeling, Perceiving)

Outgoing, friendly, and accepting. Exuberant lovers of life, people, and material comforts. Enjoy working with others to make things happen. Bring common sense and a realistic approach to their work, and make work fun. Flexible and spontaneous, adapt readily to new people and environments. Learn best by trying a new skill with other people.

ENFP (Extroversion, Intuition, Feeling, Perceiving)

Warmly enthusiastic and imaginative. See life as full of possibilities. Make connections between events and information very quickly, and confidently proceed based on the patterns they see. Want a lot of affirmation from others, and readily give appreciation and support. Spontaneous and flexible, often rely on their ability to improvise and their verbal fluency.

ENTP (Extroversion, Intuition, Thinking, Perceiving)

Quick, ingenious, stimulating, alert, and outspoken. Resourceful in solving new and challenging problems. Adept at generating conceptual possibilities and then analyzing them strategically. Good at reading other people. Bored by routine, will seldom do the same thing the same way, apt to turn to one new interest after another.

ESTJ (Extroversion, Sensing, Thinking, Judging)

Practical, realistic, matter-of-fact. Decisive, quickly move to implement decisions. Organize projects and people to get things done, focus on getting results in the most efficient way possible. Take care of routine details. Have a clear set of logical standards, systematically follow them and want others to also. Forceful in implementing their plans.

(continues)

ESFJ (Extroversion, Sensing, Feeling, Judging)

Warm hearted, conscientious, and cooperative. Want harmony in their environment, work with determination to establish it. Like to work with others to complete tasks accurately and on time. Loyal, follow through even in small matters. Notice what others need in their day-by-day lives and try to provide it. Want to be appreciated for who they are and for what they contribute.

ENFJ (Extroversion, Intuition, Feeling, Judging)

Warm, empathetic, responsive, and responsible. Highly attuned to the emotions, needs, and motivations of others. Find potential in everyone, want to help others fulfill their potential. May act as catalysts for individual and group growth. Loyal, responsive to praise and criticism. Sociable, facilitate others in a group, and provide inspiring leadership.

ENTJ (Extroversion, Intuition, Thinking, Judging)

Frank, decisive, assume leadership readily. Quickly see illogical and inefficient procedures and policies, develop and implement comprehensive systems to solve organizational problems. Enjoy long-term planning and goal setting. Usually well informed, well read, enjoy expanding their knowledge and passing it on to others. Forceful in presenting their ideas.

Contingency and Situational Theories and Leadership Styles

Contingency and situational theories postulate that effective leaders use a combination of behaviors or styles that are contingent upon the particular situation, the personalities involved, the task, and the organizational culture (Fiedler, 1967; Hersey, 1985). Contingency and situational theorists such as Fiedler (1978) and Hersey and Blanchard (1976, 1982) refrained from describing an ideal leadership style based solely on traits or personality and emphasized that successful leaders are able to understand their motivations and preferred style and are able to adapt their style to the situation and the needs of the group. Fiedler's (1978) basic premise was that leadership was a function of the leader's motivational style and the control requirements of the situation. According to the contingency theory, leaders have two primary motivations:

relationship building and task completion. In addition, the control requirements of situations depend on leader–member relations, task structure, and positional power. Leader–member relations pertain to the way followers feel about the leader. Tasks can be clearly structured or ambiguous and unstructured. Disinfecting equipment in the physical therapy clinic after a patient treatment session is an example of a highly structured task, while creating a process that will improve patient care in a particular unit from intake to exit would be considered an unstructured task.

Positional power refers to the assigned power the leader has over the group. A leader has more positional power if everyone formally reports to that leader. The attending physician has strong positional power over a group of medical residents, while a case manager has less positional power over the nurses and therapists who are part of a treatment team since each of the members report to different units in the organization.

Stress and anxiety increases when the leader's style does not match a situation, and poor decision-making is often the result. The most successful outcomes occur when leaders' preferred style matches the situational requirements and they are able to expand their behavioral repertoire through formal training. Relationship-oriented leaders are able to incorporate task-oriented behaviors, while task-oriented leaders demonstrate increased relationship-building behaviors (Fiedler, 1978; Northouse, 2010).

Hersey and Blanchard's situational theory (1976, 1982) posits that the best leaders are able shift their focus over time from task to relationships based on the developmental needs of the group. Newly formed or immature groups

that have yet to build commitment and expertise may do best with a directive, task-oriented leader, while moderately mature and mature groups are most successful when guided by a supportive, relationship-oriented leader. Ultimately, the level of engagement, participation, autonomy, and maturity that is achieved by the group depends, in part, on the degree to which decision-making authority is shared between the leader and the group members (Blanchard et al., 1985).

Blake and Mouton (1978, 1980, 1982) proposed that leadership style is informed by the degree to which the individual is concerned with task completion or relationship building. Their leadership grid (**Figure 4.1**) provided a graphic representation of the variations in leadership styles ranging from (1,1) apathetic

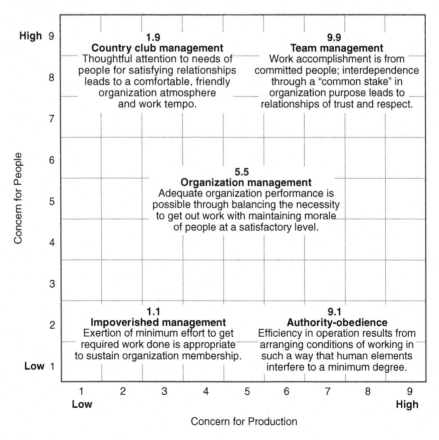

Figure 4.1 The leadership grid.

Reproduced from Blake, R., & Moulton, J. (1964). *The managerial grid: The key to leadership excellence.* Gulf Publishing Company.

REFLECTION: Blake and Mouton's Leadership Grid™

The following grid is based on the work of Blake and Mouton (1978, 1980, 1982) and depicts managerial style based on the level of caring about people (concern for people) and caring about getting the job done (concern for production).

1. In the culture of your organization, which style is the most common?
2. Is this style effective? Why or why not?

---

and not concerned with people or outcomes to (9,9) a leader who demonstrates his/her dual concern for relationship and goal attainment by fostering teamwork. Blake and Mouton identified the latter as the ideal leadership style.

Relational Theories

Later theories recognized leadership as a reciprocal interaction between leaders and followers with the hallmark of good leadership being transformation of the followers who are committed to the leader's vision (Bass & Avolio, 1994). The application of neuropsychological and neurocognitive research to the field of leadership has supplemented the wealth of information from the sociopsychological fields. Most recently, leadership is conceptualized as a set of learnable attitudes, behaviors, and skills geared toward relationship building. The effect on others is an awakening of self-efficacy, confidence, and capability, which enables proactive, engaged collective action toward a common goal (Goleman et al., 2002).

Emotional Intelligence

Decades of neuropsychological research have established that emotions can dictate our thinking, motivate us, and mobilize us into action. It is generally accepted that thoughts can induce emotions, and emotions also generate thoughts. For instance, when an individual is upset about something (emotion), he or she may engage in self-talk or internal dialogue (thoughts), which may fuel a spiral of intense emotions and upsetting thoughts.

The thoughts and emotions that shape human behavior originate from separate centers of the brain and are interactive determinants of one another. The amygdala or the feeling mind is a primitive part of the brain that triggers a fight-or-flight response, which is tempered by the prefrontal cortex or thinking mind. When stress, drugs, or alcohol compromises the nervous system, the tempering function of the prefrontal cortex may fail to block the instructions from the amygdala, and behavior that is not rational or adaptive to the situation may result.

Effective leaders are not as susceptible to this "amygdala hijack" as other leaders are. They are tuned in to their emotional skills and are able to use them in an appropriate way and in the proper context (Goleman et al., 2004). Daniel Goleman found that outstanding leaders were judged by their superiors as performing significantly better on a constellation of personal skills and social skills that fell into the following four broad categories: self-awareness, self-management, social awareness, and relationship management. This constellation of behaviors has been termed emotional intelligence (**Table 4.3**) and is a prerequisite for relationship building that is the bedrock of sustainable leadership practices (Goleman, 1995). Developing competency in relationship management is contingent upon competency in self-awareness, self-management, and social awareness and is essential for success in life and/or the workplace.

In most healthcare organizations, leaders and managers are often appointed based on expertise and years of experience. However, as supervisory responsibility increases, so does the need for people-handling skills. Research indicates that some leaders and managers who

Table 4.3 Emotional Intelligence Domains

Self-Awareness: The ability of an individual to be cognizant of his/her own emotions, acknowledge personal strengths and weaknesses, and describe how emotions impact his/her actions. Self-awareness includes the emotional self-awareness competency and is highly correlated with accurate self-assessment and self-confidence.

Self-Management: The ability to moderate negative emotional responses, to remain calm in stressful situations, adapt to change, continually work to improve oneself, and stay optimistic in challenging situations. Competencies include achievement orientation, adaptability, emotional self-control, and positive outlook.

Social Awareness: The ability to understand other individuals, teams, and organizations by being open to other perspectives, putting oneself in another person's shoes, and understanding the values, culture, and unspoken rules in a team or organization. The competencies included are empathy and organizational awareness.

Relationship Management: The ability to constructively resolve conflicts, coach and mentor others, inspire others by expressing a compelling vision, strategically influence others, and work as an effective member of a team. These competencies include skills in conflict management, coaching and mentoring, influencing, inspirational leadership, and team building.

Adapted from Goleman, D., Boyatzis, R., & McKee, A. (2002). *Primal leadership: Realizing the power of emotional intelligence.* Harvard Business School Press.

are appointed primarily because of technical skill may lack the necessary emotional and relational competencies that enable them to lead and/or manage effectively (Goleman et al., 2004). They also need personal and social skills, which are the bases for emotional intelligence and are essential for effective leadership. In a team environment, skills such as effective listening, adaptability, empathy, collaboration, and the ability to give and use feedback are requisite for not only the designated leader, but for all members of the team. When members of a team are emotionally intelligent, they can create a collaborative atmosphere that leverages the inherent skills and power of the whole group (Goleman et al., 2002).

REFLECTION: Emotional Intelligence Checklist

Rate yourself on each of the components of the emotional intelligence checklist to determine your characteristics in each of the domains.

Emotional Intelligence Checklist	
SELF-AWARENESS	
Emotional self-awareness: Recognizing how our emotions affect our performance	One who has emotional self-awareness: ■ Is aware of one's own feelings and can speak openly about them ■ Can identify the triggers to and inner signals of his or her own emotions ■ Recognizes the effects of one's own feelings on one's behavior ■ Displays emotional insight, seeing the big picture in a complex situation

(continues)

REFLECTION: Emotional Intelligence Checklist   *(continued)*

Accurate self-assessment: Knowing one's own inner resources, abilities, and limits	One who makes an accurate self-assessment: ■ Is aware of his or her own strengths and limitations ■ Welcomes honest, constructive criticism and is open to feedback ■ Has a sense of humor about oneself ■ Knows when to seek assistance
Self-confidence: A strong sense of one's self-worth and capabilities	One who has self-confidence: ■ Is confident in his or her job capability ■ Knows one's own strengths and believes in his or her own abilities ■ Displays a self-assurance that is visible to others ■ Has presence

SELF-MANAGEMENT

Emotional self-control: Keeping disruptive emotions and impulses in check	One who has emotional self-control: ■ Does not act impulsively ■ Does not get impatient or show frustration ■ Behaves calmly in stressful situations ■ Stays composed and positive, even in trying moments
Transparency: Maintaining integrity, acting congruently with one's values	One who exhibits transparency: ■ Keeps promises ■ Addresses unethical behavior in others ■ Openly and publicly admits to mistakes ■ Lives and acts on values
Adaptability: Flexibility in handling change	One who is adaptable: ■ Adapts ideas based on new information ■ Applies standard procedures flexibly ■ Handles unexpected demands well ■ Changes overall strategy, goals, or projects to fit the situation
Achievement: Striving to improve or meeting a standard of excellence	One who exhibits achievement: ■ Seeks ways to improve performance ■ Sets measurable and challenging goals ■ Anticipates obstacles to a goal ■ Takes calculated risks to reach a goal
Initiative: Readiness to act on opportunities	One who has initiative: ■ Does not hesitate to act on opportunities ■ Seeks information in unusual ways ■ Cuts through red tape and bends rules when necessary ■ Initiates actions to create possibilities
Optimism: Persistence in pursuing goals despite obstacles and setbacks	One who has optimism: ■ Has mainly positive expectations ■ Believes the future will be better than the past ■ Stays positive despite setbacks ■ Learns from setbacks

SOCIAL AWARENESS

Empathy: Sensing others' feelings and perspectives and taking an active interest in their concerns	One who has empathy: ▪ Listens attentively ▪ Is attentive to people's moods or nonverbal cues ▪ Relates well to people of diverse backgrounds ▪ Can see things from someone else's perspective
Organizational awareness: Reading a group's emotional currents and power relationships	One who has organizational awareness: ▪ Is able to detect crucial social networks and key power relationships ▪ Understands political forces within the organization ▪ Identifies the organization's guiding values ▪ Recognizes unspoken rules of the organization
Service: Anticipating, recognizing, and meeting customers' or clients' needs	One who provides service: ▪ Makes him/herself available as needed ▪ Monitors client satisfaction ▪ Fosters an environment that keeps client relationships on the right track ▪ Ensures that client needs are met

RELATIONSHIP MANAGEMENT

Inspirational leadership: Inspiring and guiding individuals and groups	One who provides inspirational leadership: ▪ Leads by example ▪ Makes work exciting ▪ Inspires others ▪ Articulates a compelling vision
Influence: Having impact on others	One who has influence: ▪ Engages an audience when presenting ▪ Persuades by appealing to people's self-interest ▪ Gets support from key people ▪ Develops behind-the-scenes support
Developing others: Sensing others' development needs and bolstering their abilities	One who develops others: ▪ Recognizes specific strengths of others ▪ Gives directions or demonstrations to develop someone ▪ Gives constructive feedback ▪ Provides ongoing mentoring or coaching
Change catalyst: Initiating or managing change	One who is a change catalyst: ▪ States need for change ▪ Is not reluctant to change or make changes ▪ Personally leads change initiatives ▪ Advocates change despite opposition
Conflict management: Negotiating and resolving conflict	One who manages conflict: ▪ Airs disagreements or conflicts ▪ Publicly states everyone's position to those involved in a conflict ▪ Does not avoid conflict ▪ Finds a position everyone can endorse

(continues)

REFLECTION: Emotional Intelligence Checklist   *(continued)*

Teamwork and collaboration: Working with others and creating group synergy in pursuing collective goals	One who exhibits teamwork and collaboration: ■ Cooperates with others ■ Solicits others' input ■ In a group, encourages others' participation ■ Establishes and maintains close relationships at work

Data from Goleman, D., Boyatzis, R., & McKee, A. (2002). *Primal leadership: Realizing the power of emotional intelligence.* Harvard Business School Press.

Resonance

The perceived attitude and emotional status of the leader is instrumental in the creation of a positive or negative emotional climate (Nembhard & Edmondson, 2006; Pescosolido, 2000). When a leader is impatient, frustrated, or fearful of failure, the group members react with defensive and self-protective behaviors—often setting off a reciprocal volley of destructive emotions and creating a dissonant and unproductive climate that is focused on self-preservation rather than co-creation. Conversely, leaders who project enthusiasm, realistic optimism, and care for the group engender these same feelings within the group. The group members are engaged, in sync, or are resonant with the leader and each other and have more energy to engage in the work of the group and face challenges more creatively (Pescosolido, 2000).

According to Boyatzis and McKee (2005), resonant leaders are mindful, compassionate, and hopeful and are skilled in eliciting affiliative and affirmative emotions in others. They are mindful in that they are fully aware of themselves, others, and the environment and are committed to their values while being open to other perspectives. The manifestation of hopefulness is confidence in their own and the group's ability to reify dreams. Compassion is reflected in their acceptance that they, in concert with their fellow humans, have strengths and vulnerabilities and are not omniscient. They face challenges and opportunities with equanimity and respect the contributions and value of the people they lead and those they serve (**Figure 4.2**).

There seems to be agreement that the best leaders are self-aware, self-regulating, and attuned to the diverse perspectives, needs, and abilities of their followers and to the requirements of the situation. Good leaders have high levels of social and emotional intelligence, an ability to develop and maintain reciprocal relationships, and a willingness to empower others, and they are able to employ a balance of task-related and relation-building behaviors. Put simply, good leaders can get the job done well while maintaining a supportive emotional atmosphere (Goleman, 1998; Kouzes & Posner, 2007; Maxwell, 2005; Whitney et al., 2010).

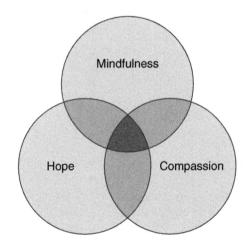

Figure 4.2 The resonant leader.

Data from Boyatzis, R., & McKee, A. (2005). *Resonant leadership.* Boston, MA: Harvard Business School Press.

References

Ashton, M., Lee, K., & de Vries, R. (2014). The HEXACO Honesty-Humility, Agreeableness, and Emotionality Factors: A review of research and theory. *Personality and Social Psychology Review, 18*, 139–152.

Avolio, B. (2007). Promoting more integrative strategies for leadership theory building. *American Psychologist, 62*, 25–33.

Bass, B. M., & Avolio, B. J. (Eds.). (1994). *Improving organizational effectiveness through transformational leadership.* Sage Publications.

Blake, R., & Moulton, J. (1964). *The managerial grid: The key to leadership excellence.* Gulf Publishing Company.

Blake, R., & Mouton, J. (1978). *The new managerial grid.* Gulf.

Blake, R., & Mouton, J. (1980). *The versatile manager: A grid profile.* Dow Jones/Irwin.

Blake, R., & Mouton, J. (1982). How to choose a leadership style. *Training and Development Journal, 36*, 39–46.

Blanchard, K., Zigarmi, P., & Zigarmi, D. (1985). *Leadership and the one minute manager.* William Morrow.

Boyatzis, R., & McKee, A. (2005). *Resonant leadership.* Harvard Business School Press.

Carlyle, T. (1841). *On heroes, hero worship and the heroic in history.* James Fraser.

Fiedler, F. (1967). *A theory of leadership effectiveness.* McGraw Hill.

Fiedler, F. (1978). The contingency model and the dynamics of the leadership process. *Advances in Experimental Social Psychology, 12*, 59–112.

Goleman, D. (1995). *Emotional intelligence.* Bantam Books.

Goleman, D. (1998). *Working with emotional intelligence.* Bantam Books.

Goleman, D., & Boyatzis, R. (2008). Social intelligence and the biology of leadership. *Harvard Business Review, 86*(9), 74–81.

Goleman, D., Boyatzis, R., & McKee, A. (2002). *Primal leadership: Realizing the power of emotional intelligence.* Harvard Business School Press.

Goleman, D., Boyatzis, R., & McKee, A. (2004). *Primal leadership: Learning to lead with emotional intelligence.* Harvard Business School Press.

Hersey, P. (1985). *The situational leader.* Warner Books.

Hersey, P., & Blanchard, K. (1976). Leader effectiveness and adaptability description (LEAD). In J. W. Pfeiffer & J. E. Jones (Eds.), *The 1976 annual handbook for group facilitators* (Vol. 5). University Associates.

Hersey, P., & Blanchard, K. (1982). *Management of organizational behavior: Utilizing human resources* (4th ed.). Prentice Hall.

Hogan, R., & Hogan, J. (2007). *Hogan personality inventory manual* (3rd ed.). Hogan Assessment Systems.

Hogan, R. & Smither, R. (2008). *Personality: Theories and applications.* Hogan Press.

Jung, C. G. (1991). *The development of personality* (Collected Works, Vol. 17). Routledge. (Original published in 1910.)

Kouzes, J., & Posner, B. (2007). *The leadership challenge.* Jossey-Bass.

Maxwell, J. C. (2005). *The 360° leader: Developing your influence from anywhere in the organization.* Nelson Business.

McCrae, R., & Costa, P. (1987). Validation of the five factor model of personality across instruments and observers. *Journal of Personality and Social Psychology, 52*, 81–90.

Myers, I. B., McCaulley, M. H., Quenk, N. L., & Hammer, A. L. (1998). *MBTI manual: A guide to the development and use of the Myers-Briggs type indicator* (3rd ed.). Consulting Psychologists Press.

Nembhard, I., & Edmondson, A. (2006). Making it safe: The effects of leader inclusiveness and professional status on psychological safety and improvement efforts in health care teams. *Journal of Organizational Behavior, 27*, 941–966.

Northouse, P. (2010). *Leadership: Theory and practice.* SAGE Publications.

Pescosolido, A. T. (2000). *The leader's emotional impact in work groups* (Doctoral dissertation). Case Western Reserve University.

Stoffel, V. (2014). Presidential address, attitude, authenticity, and action: Building capacity. *American Journal of Occupational Therapy, 68*, 628–635. http://dx.doi.org/10.5014/ajot.2014.686002

Tolstoy, L. (2010). *War and peace* (New edition). Oxford University Press. (Original work published in 1867.)

Whitney, D., Trosten-Bloom, A., & Radu, K. (2010). *Appreciative leadership: Focus on what works to drive winning performance.* McGraw Hill.

Zaccaro, S. (2007). Trait based perspectives of leadership. *American Psychologist, 62*, 6–16.

CHAPTER 5

Leadership Building Blocks

LEARNING OBJECTIVES

1. Describe the uses of power and authority.
2. Assess leader behaviors and how they relate to power.
3. Define motivation and how it affects leadership styles.
4. Describe how adult learning and learning preferences affect leadership behaviors.
5. Explain the relationship of self-directed learning and personal transformation.

The most recent thinking on leadership recognizes an interaction between traits, styles, context, and social dynamics. Good leaders can reflect on their own behavior and evaluate their personal strengths, weaknesses, biases, needs, and motivations. The honest appraisal of their own gifts and vulnerabilities engenders empathy for the gifts and vulnerabilities of others. This appreciation of the perspective of others facilitates a collaborative attitude that engages and inspires peers and subordinates to action.

The study of how leadership has evolved and the requisite knowledge, skills, and attitudes for effective leadership can be organized into three broad categories: power, motivation, and learning.

Power

In the 1960s classic on management, *The Human Side of Enterprise*, Douglas McGregor examined the effects of leading/managing behaviors on subordinates using the theory X and theory Y approaches. In summary, theory X contends that employees are motivated mainly by money and must be controlled, directed, and threatened with punishment in order to work toward the achievement of organizational objectives. Theory Y, on the other hand, focuses on the creation of an environment that rewards the exercise of initiative, ingenuity, and self-direction and views opportunities for engagement and self-actualization as motivating forces. Leaders will often speak about their beliefs and philosophies of leadership as if they are aligned with theory Y. Their actions, however, are often more reflective of theory X. Research has shown that inviting participation, facilitating positive group and employee manager interaction, and giving workers responsibility improve productivity. Despite this research, theory X still informs many management decisions (Ryan & Deci, 2000; Spreier et al., 2006). The command-and-control aspect of theory X is attractive because it may yield short-term results. However, the social capital, engagement, loyalty, and sustained productivity that are associated with theory Y may be sacrificed (Spreitzer & Porath, 2012; Edmondson, 2019).

The exercise of authority is necessary for a group to form and develop. In other words, someone needs to step up to the plate to get the ball rolling. However, in order for groups to mature, power and authority have to be distributed evenly over time. The distribution of authority and power in groups is as much a function of a person's position in the organization as it is the perception that group members have of that person. In the absence of specific information to the contrary, group members will attribute high or low status and related power and authority to individuals based on certain physical characteristics (height, strength), gender, race, ethnicity, or professional association (physician, professor, lawyer) (Berger et al., 1972). Six categories of power have been defined: referent, legitimate, expertise, coercion, reward, and informational. Referent power means that power is inferred through explicit status or personal characteristics such as charm or decisiveness. For example, team members make an assumption that the physician will be a leader since being a physician is considered a high-status position. Legitimate power resides with the person, such as a chief executive officer (CEO), who, by nature of the position, wields power. Expert power belongs to those who have specialized knowledge, information, and skills. Coercive power relates to the ability to distribute negative consequences, such pay cuts or demotions, while reward power addresses the ability to offer positive incentives, such as pay raises and promotions. Information power is based on the access to information that is valued by others. As the access to valued information increases, so does the power to provide rational arguments and influence decision making (French & Raven, 1959; Raven, 2008).

Power and status differentials are a fact of life and frequently limit the participation of team members who perceive themselves to be of lower status. Limitations in participation are often related to reduced engagement in the group process along with diminished accountability for group outcomes. If this disengagement is experienced by team members who do not hold high-status positions, the team will not benefit from their expertise, and the team will not have the cohesion necessary to reach its functional potential (Edmondson, 2019; Eppich et al., 2016). Research suggests that in groups without a designated leader, power is given in the form of attention to the individuals who are the most emotionally expressive and who have

---

REFLECTION: **Who's Got the Power?**

If a CEO, a physician, and a sailor were on a storm-tossed ship, who do you think would be the most powerful of the three? What kind of power does he/she have?

Suppose the CEO, physician, and sailor land safely on a remote island that houses a secret military base. They are mistaken for spies and taken to the base commander who will determine their fate. Describe how the commander might exercise coercive power.

the most valued traits (Goleman, 2011). These assumptions, in combination with the traditional medical hierarchy and actual differences in disciplinary cultures, professional education, experience, and responsibility, contribute to the variations in dominance, prestige, and control in healthcare teams. The literature is replete with examples of how the traditional hierarchies in healthcare practices have proved detrimental to the harnessing of the power of the collective intelligence that exists among diverse groups of healthcare workers (Drinka & Clark, 2000; Freshman et al., 2010; Garman et al., 2006; Gittell, 2009; Gray, 2008; Institute of Medicine, 2001, 2003; Lee, 2010).

Leaders can mitigate the effects of status and power differentials on group participation by employing *co-creative power* and making a conscious effort to create a psychologically safe atmosphere where inclusive participation is the norm (Nembhard & Edmondson, 2006; Edmondson, 2019). *Co-creative power* leverages interconnectedness and facilitates the collective intelligence of the group. *Co-creative power* is a term that was coined by Mary Parker Follett early in the twentieth century and is inherent to concepts such as participatory management, quality circles, and distributed leadership in groups. Her ideas are consistent with systems theory and the integrative, reflective practices that are considered hallmarks of learning organizations, successful agents of change, and innovative groups (Briskin et al., 2009; Pype et al., 2018; Tannenbaum & Cerasoli, 2013; Sampath et al., 2021).

Power over is a traditional relationship in which one person has power over another person or one group over another group…It is a relationship of polarity. *Power with* is at once relational and collective…an organizational form of collaboration…*co-creative power. Power with* has the boldness to believe that acting from immediate self-interest is not always the wisest course of action, nor that one person or one group should be in a position to know what is best for the other. (Briskin et al., 2009, p. 94)

It is understood that power can arise from an individual's personal characteristics or social status (referent power), position (legitimate power), specialized skill (expert power), ability to distribute rewards or punishment (reward/coercive power), or access to information (informational power) (French & Raven, 1959; Raven, 2008). Some individuals possess all six sources of power by virtue of their status and personal magnetism, designated position in the organization, expertise, and ability to dispense rewards and punishment. Does this make them influential and effective leaders? You would have to examine how the person exercised power and what effect it had on the followers before you could judge his or her success as a leader. How transformational and sustainable was his or her effect on others' behavior? Did the followers merely do as they were told or did they internalize the leader's message and move forward inspired by a mission?

REFLECTION: Power Assessment

Identify two individuals who you think are powerful.
List the specific behaviors each of them uses in exercising that power.
What type of power are they using?
Is one individual more effective than the other? Why?
Could you see yourself using power in the same way?
Why? Why not?

Motivation

David McClelland (1953, 1987) hypothesized that human behavior is a result of a complex mix of motivations—some of which are stronger than others. McClelland found that most behavior can be organized into three social motives or needs: achievement orientation, affiliation, and power. Achievement orientation describes the drive to attain challenging goals and exceed personal expectation for results. People with a high achievement orientation enjoy achieving their own personal best. People with dominant achievement orientation tend to like jobs where they can succeed based on their expertise. Affiliation describes the need for friendly and close relationships, so people with high affiliation prefer to work with others and value harmony and collaboration. People with a high affiliation motive also tend to value harmonious relationships over achievement and power and will do whatever they can in the workplace to preserve relationships. Power motive describes the need to be in charge or strongly influence another person's or group's behavior. People who have a high power motive tend to want their ideas to prevail and are interested in increasing personal status and prestige.

Power motive is often misunderstood as a negative trait. Yukl (1989) differentiates between personal power and socialized power. People with highly personalized power may have little inhibition or self-control, and they exercise power impulsively. When they give advice or support, it is with strategic intent to further bolster their own status. They demand loyalty to themselves rather than to the organization. The result is often disorder and breakdown of team morale and direction that takes place behind the leader's back. Socialized power need is most often associated with effective leadership. These leaders direct their need for power in socially positive ways that benefit others and the organization rather than only contributing to the leader's status and

gain. They seek power because it is through power that tasks are accomplished. They recognize that power must be distributed and shared and that other people need to have power over their own work lives. Effective leaders empower others who use that power to enact and further the leader's vision for the organization.

McClelland (1953, 1987) hypothesized that the most successful leaders appear to be driven mainly by a high achievement orientation, in combination with a need to empower others and forge relationships. Further research yielded that primary motivating factors informed specific leadership behavioral styles, such as directive, pacesetting, visionary, affiliative, participative, and coaching styles. Exclusive use of any one style can lead to unintended, negative consequences. For instance, highly directive and pacesetting leaders may micromanage and focus on goals rather than people, which can lead to demoralized and disengaged teams. Leaders who are myopic in their attention to relationship building may avoid giving negative feedback, avoid confrontation, and worry so much about people that they lose their ability to objectively evaluate performance. Leaders who had a repertoire of visionary, affiliative, participative, and coaching behaviors created energizing work climates, but those who were primarily pacesetting tended to create neutral or demotivating work climates. The most effective leaders are those who have a curiosity and respect for their own and others' needs, motivation, strengths, weaknesses, and preferred modes of learning (**Table 5.1**). Effective leaders also have an ability to adjust their style to fit the situation in order to facilitate positive outcomes (Spreier et al., 2006; Goleman, 2000).

A tool that is used for self-discovery and leadership development is the Fundamental Interpersonal Relations Orientation (FIRO) (Schutz, 1958). The FIRO is based on the theory that there are three primary motivating factors for individuals' behavior in

Table 5.1 Leadership Style Summary

Leadership Style	Focus	Purpose
Directive	Moving toward immediate action, give clear directions	Decisive action in emergency situations
Visionary	Clear communication, move people toward shared dreams	Provide redirection for change initiatives
Affiliative	Harmonious relationships	Bridge building and motivation during stressful times
Participative	Consensus building, engagement, and commitment	Developing collective buy-in
Pacesetting	Meeting challenges	Achieving high-quality results with highly competent team
Coaching	Development and mentoring of others	Building long-term team and organizational capabilities

Data from Spreier, S. W., Fontaine, M. H., & Malloy, R. L. (2006). Leadership run amok: The destructive potential of overachievers. *Harvard Business Review*, *84*(6), 72–82.

groups: inclusion, control, and affection. People who are motivated primarily by the need for inclusion will tend to be very social and interactive. Those who are driven by the need to control might be autocratic in their dealings with others, while those who have a strong desire to be liked may spend a great deal of time developing strong relationships.

Measurements from the FIRO and the Myers-Briggs Type Indicators (MBTI) are highly correlated and are often used together to provide a typology for assessing the primary motivating factors for a leader's behaviors and the preferred behavioral style. These assessments are used for self-discovery and learning and are not designed to be used for evaluative purposes.

Learning

Self-awareness and the ability to consider the impact of interactive and learning styles on group function and to change accordingly are hallmarks of transformational learning and effective leadership (Goleman, 1995; Hersey & Blanchard, 1976, 1982; Whitney

et al., 2010). Successful healthcare team leaders and members must navigate multiple relationships, be open to new ideas, solve complex problems, and generate innovative and effective solutions. Adjusting, adapting, and innovating are all, in essence, outcomes of learning (Brown & Posner, 2001; Vaill, 1998; Sampath et al., 2021). Leadership is a developmental process that can be viewed as a lifelong journey that incorporates the cognitive (what you learn) and metacognitive (how you learn) aspects of learning. An understanding of adult learning theories and their relationship to the development of leadership behaviors will help healthcare team members to adapt and thrive in complex healthcare environments.

Andragogy—the study of adult learning—posits that over time, humans develop fixed ideas, which are cognitive structures or fixed gestalts regarding themselves and the world around them. Learning happens when an individual's established ideas are challenged through experience or conflicting external forces (Knowles et al., 2005). The literature regarding learning and leadership corroborates andragogy's premise. Leaders tend to learn best when learning is self-directed, transformational, and experiential (Brown & Posner, 2001; Dalton, 1999; Kouzes & Posner, 2007; Mirriam et al., 2007; Zemke, 1985).

Self-directed learning means that adult learners need to be autonomous in what they learn, when they learn, and how they learn. Adults must be given enough information and background to understand why they should take the time to learn something new. Learning activities must be interactive, adaptable to differing learning styles, and applicable to real-life situations.

Mezirow (1981) identified an individual's overall worldview as "meaning perspective" that is generated in childhood and composed of values, beliefs, and experiences. Meaning perspectives serve as perceptual filters and determine how an individual will organize and interpret the meaning of his/her life's experiences. When schemas are disrupted by new experiences, information, traumatic life events, ideas, or concepts, transformational learning takes place and alters our view on the micro and macro levels (Clarke, 1993; Mezirow, 1981; Mirriam et al., 2007). Inherent to this perceptual shift is the realization that individuals can explore new behaviors and liberate their power as agents of change rather than victims of change. This personal transformation increases self-efficacy and the confidence to employ leadership behaviors to impact not only personal growth but also change and growth in the people and groups outside of oneself (Friere, 1973).

Adults learn best when they can engage in experiential learning and employ the wisdom of past experiences when meeting new challenges. Leaders will almost always cite trial-and-error experiences rather than formal coursework as their most pivotal learning events (Bryan, 2011).

Kolb (1974, 2015) developed a cyclical model of adult learning that describes four primary learning modes: concrete experiences (CE), reflective observations (RO), abstract conceptualizations (AC), and active experimentation (AE); and four combination learning modes: assimilation, accommodation, converging, and diverging. According to this model, the most valuable adult learning experiences are characterized by opportunities to act, reflect on action, obtain feedback on action, make sense of the experience, and engage in active experimentation of alternative actions (**Figure 5.1**). The Kolb Learning Style Inventory (KLSI4.0) (2015) is a self-report questionnaire that identifies four primary learning modes, four combination learning modes, and nine distinctive learning styles that emphasize either one of the primary learning modes, a convergence of two of the primary learning modes, or a balance of all four of the primary learning modes (**Table 5.2**).

Convergers have high scores in the AC and AE areas and like to engage in the practical application of theories to solve specific problems. Divergers have high scores in CE and RO. They are imaginative and creative and like to see situations from many perspectives. Assimilators score highest in the AC and RO areas and excel in developing theoretical concepts. Accommodators score highest in the CE and AE areas and prefer risk-taking and solving problems in a collaborative, trial-and-error fashion.

In addition to tools such as the FIRO, MBTI-measurements such as the Kolb LSI serve to further expand self-knowledge. In short, the Kolb inventory provides a method for understanding whether one learns best by trial and error, developing theory, applying theory to practice, or collaborating with others (**Table 5.3**). In addition to broadening a potential leader's self-knowledge, these tools also serve as a point of reference when trying to comprehend and influence the behavior of others. A leader has a much better chance of understanding and influencing others when their interests and perspectives are addressed.

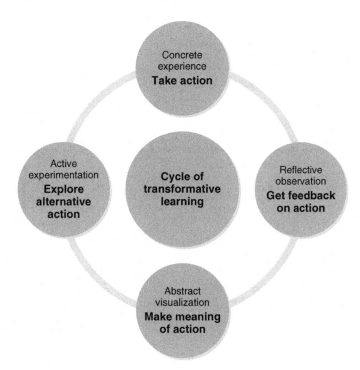

Figure 5.1 Kolb model of adult learning.

Based on Kolb, D. (1974). On management and the learning process. In D. Kolb, I. Rubin, & J. McIntyre (Eds.), *Organizational psychology: A book of readings* (pp. 27–42). Prentice Hall.

Table 5.2 Kolb Learning Modes Summary

Primary Learning Modes	
Concrete Experience (CE)	Abstract Conceptualization (AC)
Active Experimentation (AE)	Reflective Observation (RO)
Combination Learning Modes	
Assimilation	Accommodation
Converging	Diverging

Data from Kolb, D. (1974). On management and the learning process. In D. Kolb, I. Rubin, & J. McIntyre (Eds.), *Organizational psychology: A book of readings* (pp. 27–42). Prentice Hall.

Table 5.3 Kolb Learner Behaviors

Concrete Experience (CE)	Learns by direct experience, discussion, and feedback from others
Reflective Observation (RO)	Learns by listening and reflecting
Abstract Conceptualization (AC)	Learns by logical thinking and objective analysis
Active Experimentation (AE)	Learns by active engagement

Data from Kolb, D. (1974). On management and the learning process. In D. Kolb, I. Rubin, & J. McIntyre (Eds.), *Organizational psychology: A book of readings* (pp. 27–42). Prentice Hall.

REFLECTION: What Type of Learner Are You?

Review **Table 5.4**. Which behaviors and attitudes most closely match yours? How do these behaviors and attitudes impact your ability to lead?

Table 5.4 Kolb Learning Styles Summary

Learning Style	Learning Modes	Learner behavior
Initiating	**Active Experimentation** **Concrete Experience**	Thinks quickly and takes risks. Seeks new opportunities. Influences others. Preference for learning in context.
Experiencing	**Concrete Experience** Active Experimentation Reflective Observation	Intuitive. Mindful. Emotionally intelligent. Enjoys relationships.
Imagining	**Concrete Experience** **Reflective Observation**	Reflective. Receptive to diverse ideas, people, experiences, and possibility.
Reflecting	**Reflective Observation** Concrete Experience Abstract Conceptualization	Connects experience and ideas through sustained reflection. Observes, takes multiple perspectives and waits to act until certain of the outcome.
Analyzing	**Reflective Observation** **Abstract Conceptualization**	Plans ahead to minimize mistakes. Integrates information to get the full picture, and uses theories and models to test assumptions.
Thinking	**Abstract Conceptualization** Active Experimentation Reflective Observation	Uses disciplined, abstract reasoning. Utilizes logic and critical thinking to analyze data and reach solutions.
Deciding	**Abstract Conceptualization** **Active Experimentation**	Sets performance goals. Evaluates progress. Selects a single course to solve problems and achieve results.
Acting	**Active Experimentation** Concrete Experience Abstract Conceptualization	Takes goal-directed action that balances accomplishments with relationships.
Balancing	**Concrete Experience** **Abstract Conceptualization** **Active Experimentation** **Reflective Observation**	Weighs the pros and cons of acting versus reflecting and experiencing versus thinking. Holistic perspective. Bridges differences and flexibly adapts to shifting priorities.

Data from SB Staff (2022, May 16). Kolb's model for experiential learning: A theory of how people learn effectively. Sounding Board Inc. Retrieved January 31, 2023, from https://www.soundingboardinc.com/blog/kolbs-model-experiential-learning-effectively/ and Learning styles. Institute for Experiential Learning. (2021, October 15). Retrieved January 31, 2023, from. https://experientiallearninginstitute.org/resources/learning-styles

---

REFLECTION: Self-Management—Mature Leader Reflection

At the heart of self-management lies an ability to reflect on one's own behavior, values, and style as well as the effect they have on others and the effect other peoples' values, behaviors, and styles have on oneself.

Mature leaders learn to do the following:

1. Stretch beyond their own personal learning style so that they can learn in every situation, even if it is not designed for their personal preference.
2. Be conscious of other people's preferred styles and adjust communication accordingly.

Answer the following questions:

3. What does your preference tell you about what you are really good at?
4. How would learning to act and work with those with opposite preferences help you be seen as a leader by others?

References

Berger, J., Cohen, P., & Zeldich, M. (1972). Status characteristics and social interaction. *American Sociological Review, 37*(3), 241–255.

Briskin, A., Erickson, S., Ott, J., & Callanan, T. (2009). *The power of collective wisdom and the trap of collective folly.* Berrett-Koehler.

Brown, L., & Posner, B. (2001). Exploring the relationship between learning and leadership. *Leadership & Organizational Development Journal, 22*(6), 274–280.

Bryan, A. (2011). *The corner office: Indispensable and unexpected lessons from CEOs on how to lead and succeed.* Times Books/Henry Holt & Co.

Clarke, M. (1993). Transformational learning. *New Directions for Adults and Continuing Education, 57,* 47–56.

Dalton, M. (1999). *The learning tactics inventory.* Jossey-Bass/Pfieffer.

Drinka, T., & Clark, P. (2000). *Health care teamwork: Interdisciplinary practice and teaching.* Auburn House.

Edmondson, A. (2019). *The fearless organization: Creating psychological safety in the workplace for learning, innovation and growth.* John Wiley & Sons.

Eppich, W., Mullan, P., Brett-Fleegler, M., & Cheng, A. (2016). "Let's Talk About It": Translating lessons from health care simulation to clinical event debriefings and coaching conversations. *Clinical Pediatric Emergency Medicine, 17*(3), 200–211.

French, J., & Raven, B. (1959). The bases of social power. In D. Cartwright & A. Zander, *Group dynamics* (pp. 259–269). Harper & Row.

Freshman, B., Rubino, L., & Chassiakos, Y. (2010). *Collaboration across the disciplines in health care.* Jones and Bartlett Publishers.

Friere, P. (1973). *Pedagogy of the oppressed.* Seabury Press.

Garman, A., Leach, D., & Spector, N. (2006). Worldviews in collision: Conflict and collaboration across professional lines. *Journal of Organizational Behaviour, 27,* 829–849.

Gittell, J. (2009). *High performance healthcare: Using the power of relationships to achieve quality, efficiency and resilience.* McGraw Hill.

Goleman, D. (1995). *Emotional intelligence.* Bantam Books.

Goleman, D. (2000). Leadership that gets results. *Harvard Business Review.*https://hbr.org/2000/03/leadership-that-gets-results

Goleman, D. (2011). *Leadership: The power of emotional intelligence.* More Than Sound.

Gray, B. (2008). Enhancing transdisciplinary research through collaborative leadership. *American Journal of Preventive Medicine, 35*(2S), s124–s132.

Hersey, P., & Blanchard, K. (1976). Leader effectiveness and adaptability description (LEAD). In J. W. Pfeiffer & J. E. Jones (Eds.), *The 1976 annual handbook for group facilitators* (Vol. 5). University Associates.

Hersey, P., & Blanchard, K. (1982). *Management of organizational behavior: Utilizing human resources* (4th ed.). Prentice Hall.

Institutes of Medicine. (2001). *Crossing the quality chasm: A new health system for the 21st century.* National Academy Press.

Institute of Medicine, Committee on Educating Public Health Professionals for the 21st Century; Gebbie, K., Rosenstock, L., & Hernandez, L. M. (Eds.). (2003). *Who will keep the public healthy? Educating public health professionals for the 21st century.* National Academies Press.

Institute of Medicine, Committee on the Health Professions Education Summit; Greiner, A. C., & Knebel, E. (Eds.). (2003). *Health professions education: A bridge to quality.* National Academies Press.

Institute of Medicine, Committee on Quality of Health Care in America. (2001). *Crossing the quality chasm: A new health system for the 21st century.* National Academies Press.

Knowles, M., Holton, E., & Swanson, R. (2005). *The adult learner: The definitive classic in adult education and human resource development* (6th ed.). Elsevier.

Kolb, D. (1974). On management and the learning process. In D. Kolb, I. Rubin, & J. McIntyre (Eds.), *Organizational psychology: A book of readings* (pp. 27–42). Prentice Hall.

Kolb, D. (2015). *Experiential learning: Experience as the source of learning and development* (2nd ed.). Pearson Education.

Kouzes, J., & Posner, B. (2007). *The leadership challenge.* Jossey-Bass.

Lee, T. H. (2010). Turning doctors into leaders. *Harvard Business Review, 88*(4), 50–58.

McClelland, D. (1953). *The achievement motive.* Appleton-Century Crofts.

McClelland, D. (1987). *Human motivation.* Cambridge University Press.

McGregor, D. (1960). *The human side of enterprise.* McGraw Hill.

Mezirow, J. (1981). A critical theory of adult learning and education. *Adult Education Quarterly, 32*(1), 3–24.

Mirriam, S., Caffarella, R., & Baumgartner, L. (2007). *Learning in adulthood: A comprehensive guide.* Jossey-Bass.

Nembhard, I., & Edmondson, A. (2006). Making it safe: The effects of leader inclusiveness and professional status on psychological safety and improvement efforts in health care teams. *Journal of Organizational Behavior, 27*, 941–966.

Pype, P., Mertens, F., Helewaut, F., & Krystallidou, D. (2018). Healthcare teams as complex adaptive systems: Understanding team behavior through team members' perception of interpersonal interaction. *BMC Health Services Research, 18*, 570. https://doi.org/10/1186/s12913-018-3392-3.

Raven, B. (2008). The bases of power and the power/interaction model of interpersonal influence. *Analysis of Social Issues and Public Policy, 8*(1), 1–22.

Ryan, R., & Deci, E. (2000). Self determination theory and the facilitation of intrinsic motivation, social development and well being. *American Psychologist, 55*, 68–78.

Sampath, B., Rakover, J., Baldoza, K., Mate, K., Lenoci-Edwards, J., & Barker, P. (2021). *Whole system quality: A unified approach to building responsive, resilient health care systems* (IHI White Paper). Institute for Healthcare Improvement.

Schutz, W. (1958). *FIRO: A three dimensional theory of interpersonal behavior.* Rinehart.

Spreier, S. W., Fontaine, M. H., & Malloy, R. L. (2006). Leadership run amok: The destructive potential of overachievers. *Harvard Business Review, 84*(6), 72–82.

Spreitzer, G., & Porath, C. (2012). Creating sustainable performance. *Harvard Business Review, 90*(1–2), 92–99.

Tannenbaum, S., & Cerasoli, C. (2013). Do team and individual debriefs enhance performance? A meta-analysis. *Human Factors, 55*(1), 231–245.

Vaill, P. (1998). *Spirited leading and learning.* Jossey-Bass.

Whitney, D., Trosten-Bloom, A., & Radu, K. (2010). *Appreciative leadership: Focus on what works to drive winning performance.* McGraw Hill.

Yukl, G. A. (1989). *Leadership in organizations.* Prentice Hall.

Zigarmi, L. (2019). *How leaders can create fearless teams.* http://www.forbes.com.sites/forbescoachescouncil/2019/05/13/?sh=23471c65549e

Zemke, R. (1985). The Honeywell studies: How managers learn to manage. *Training, 22*(8), 46–51.

CHAPTER 6

Relational Leadership

LEARNING OBJECTIVES

1. Apply relational skills such as respect, empathy, altruism, and self-awareness to leadership.
2. Identify a personal leadership style and construct a personal philosophy of leadership.
3. Explain how assuming roles such as coach, partner, and catalyst can enhance effective leadership.
4. Evaluate the effect of personal leadership behaviors on oneself and other members of the team.
5. Use reflection and inquiry to facilitate personal and group development.

Members of the healthcare professions are well schooled in mindfulness, hope, and compassion—as applied to their relationships with their patients. Compassion and empathy for others are often the motivation for pursuing a healthcare career. Hope—the firm belief in the capability of the health professions and the resilience of the human spirit to overcome adversity and positively affect the quality of patients' lives—lies at the very core of every health profession. Good clinical reasoning requires focused examination of objective clinical information in combination with mindful, in-the-moment analysis of the complex and unique illness experience of each patient. The challenge for leaders and members of healthcare teams is to understand that it is their responsibility to employ these qualities not only with their patients but also in their interactions with coworkers, superiors, and subordinates. In addition to the development of their professional disciplinary practice, leaders and members of interprofessional healthcare teams must hone their relational leadership practice (Trezciak & Mazzarelli, 2019). Zolno (2007) perceives leadership as a relational act that is facilitated by a personal sense of self-worth, hope, and capability. Individuals who develop their own sense of worth and hope, can, through the building of positive relationships, transmit those values to others. Zolno and Skillman (2011) further describe leadership as a multifaceted action that is generative, affirmative, collaborative, catalytic, and harmonizing (**Table 6.1**). Each of these terms address the relational nature of leadership and provides a framework for examining the roles that leaders must assume in order to become agents of positive change and growth in themselves and others (Anchor, 2012).

Table 6.1 Multifaceted Leadership as Described by Zolno and Skillman

Attitude	Role	Skill
Generative	Learner	Comfortable with not knowing, openness to new learning, ability to solicit feedback from all constituencies, learn from experience, and apply knowledge to new situations
Affirmative	Coach	Ability to focus on strengths, successes, positive intentions, and potential of others; ability to broaden the perceptions of others in order to formulate new behavioral choices
Collaborative	Partner	Create an inclusive atmosphere where all ideas are welcomed and valued
Catalytic	Catalyst	Leverage diversity of thought, encourage exploration outside the box, challenge the status quo
Harmonizing	Ecologist	Ability to understand and capitalize on the interactive and interdependent nature of social systems

Data from Zolno, S., & Skillman, R. (2011). *Coaching certification in whole system IQ and appreciative inquiry.* The Leading Clinic.

The Leader as Learner

The highly specialized training that is the hallmark of traditional health professional education places a premium on knowing and leaves little room for understanding the perspectives of multiple disciplines. Those professionals who have a negative capability or an ability to "not know" are more comfortable working in the ambiguous space between disciplines and are more likely to encourage innovative thought and creative solutions to complex problems (Hammick et al., 2009; Whitney et al., 2010; Holmes, 2015). Leaders who are comfortable with ambiguity are curious about different perspectives and are open to, rather than threatened by, new ways of looking at problems and situations. By eliciting diverse perspectives, leaders broaden their own knowledge base and encourage all the members of their teams to engage in collaborative, creative problem-solving (French et al., 2001; Briskin et al., 2009).

The Leader as Coach

Coaching can be defined as the building of deep relationships in order to equip people with the knowledge, skills, and attitudes that will help them achieve their potential (Peterson & Hicks, 1996). By increasing the self-efficacy of others, the coaching leader helps to broaden their perceived range of choices and possibilities for action. The core of the coaching process is informed by andragogy or adult learning theory, which assumes that the most meaningful learning experiences for adults are experiential, self-directed, and personally relevant (Knowles et al., 2005). Kolb (1974) described adult learning as a cycle that includes concrete experiences, reflective observations, abstract conceptualizations, and active experimentation. In a coaching environment, people are encouraged to attend to how they feel about an action, reflect on that experience, make sense out of the experience, and then explore a better way to take action next time.

The designated leader of the team actively coaches team members by learning to listen, learning to ask powerful questions, and creating a safe environment based on trust and confidentiality. The leader of healthcare teams has a unique challenge in that he/she must be able to navigate between the traditional expert/novice model—"the sage on the stage"—of supervision/teaching,

CASE STORY | I Don't Know What You Are Talking About

We need to have a more robust acknowledgment about the fact that we don't know how to run an interdisciplinary/interprofessional team. We pretend we all know how it works. We are embarrassed that we don't know how to do it. I don't know that people even know what interprofessional teamwork means.

I noticed that when teams were meeting and people gave their perspective, they were using shorthand. If you were in another discipline, you didn't know what they were saying. As a nurse, I didn't understand what the occupational therapist was saying, and the social worker didn't know what the nurse was saying. Everyone nodded their heads though, thinking that they were supposed to understand. It was like we are back in grade school, and we don't want to admit that we don't

know. After the meeting, people would confide in me that "I really had no idea what so and so was saying." I started to send a message in the organization that you should assume no one knows what you are talking about unless they are in your discipline. I started to help people recognize that we cannot use shorthand language in interdisciplinary teams. I suggested that people create a template for their own shorthand and be more aware that everyone doesn't understand it and be willing to say, "I don't know what you are talking about," if they don't know what someone is talking about.

—Kevin Hook, Chief Nursing Officer, LIFE Practice, School of Nursing, University of Pennsylvania, Philadelphia, PA

REFLECTION: Lifelong Learning

Leader and Members as Lifelong Learners

Who do I want to be?	
Who am I now?	
How will I use my strengths to achieve my goals?	
Who will help me to achieve my goals?	

---

which requires the transmission of professional expertise and the "guide on the side" ability to engage others in active self-exploration and growth (McKee et al., 2009). A successful coaching relationship will create an atmosphere of respect and trust that will enable team members to assume a leadership stance and will allow them to offer their unique professional perspective while maintaining an active curiosity and actively soliciting the same from other team members. It has been suggested that coaching with compassion—helping others achieve their goals—triggers parasympathetic activity and actually counteracts the physiological and psychological effects of stress associated with positions of power (Boyatzis et al., 2006; Seppala et al., 2014).

A case manager has been experiencing difficulty getting her team to work together efficiently. She comes to her weekly session with her supervisor to discuss how she should handle this challenge. Her supervisor assumes a coaching stance and responds to the case manager's concerns:

- Can you tell me about interdisciplinary teams that have been really successful? (Concrete experience)
- Why were they successful? (Abstract conceptualization)
- What did you do to make the team successful? (Reflective observation)
- What did the members do? (Reflective observation)
- What can you do to make it more effective? (Active experimentation)

The Leader as Partner

A psychologically safe work environment mitigates the risk associated with behaviors that bridge status differentials, such as suggesting new procedures, offering unsolicited feedback, or sharing innovative ideas. Senior team members (those who hold high-status positions as well as those who have been on the job longest) have a unique opportunity to help new team members by modeling relationship-building behaviors that facilitate interpersonal trust, respect, and active engagement in collaborative team efforts. As the tenure of team members within a position increases, so does their communication and tendency to pay less attention to status differentials. As status barriers fade and team-wide collaboration increases, opportunities for creative problem solving and innovation abound. A key component of leadership development initiatives is learning how to be inclusive and to foster psychological safety within

healthcare teams because this is linked to quality improvement in patient care (Nembhard & Edmondson, 2006).

The Leader as Catalyst

The focus on building relationships in order to empower others to act rather than the exercise of control over the actions of others is synonymous with the concept of servant leadership and particularly cogent to teams of health professionals. Servant leaders appreciate and leverage the expertise and contributions of every member of the healthcare team in order to enhance patient outcomes (Hammick et al., 2009; Neill et al., 2007). Knowing when to defer to the expertise of others is a valuable trait for leaders/members of interprofessional healthcare teams. The strength of the team lies in its ability to leverage the skills of multiple disciplines toward the common goal of client-centered care. While individual members of the interprofessional team have a comfort level with traditionally prescribed roles and responsibilities, they must be cognizant of the limits of their knowledge and capabilities and reach beyond disciplinary boundaries in order to facilitate relationships and client-centered versus disciplinary-centered practice.

The Leader as Ecologist

With specialized training comes greater natural resistance to new methods and approaches and difficulty communicating those approaches across disciplines. Bridging the gaps between disciplines is a key role healthcare leaders can play for their organization (Garman, 2010). By listening actively and asking questions rather than making statements, leaders/members of healthcare teams can cross disciplinary boundaries. They can move from conflict to learning and status quo to innovation in relationship-based, patient-centered care (French et al., 2001; Gray, 2008; Klein, 2010).

It appears that the most effective leaders are those who can focus attention on group goals and the orientation of others. Gray (2008) suggests that leadership behaviors in well-functioning interdisciplinary groups can be categorized by cognitive, structural, and procedural tasks. Cognitive tasks often take the form of appreciative forms of inquiry where the focus is placed on how the team can make best practice the norm rather than how the team can avoid mistakes. Establishing strong social networks within the team and with stakeholders outside of the team are structural or bridge-building behaviors that serve to neutralize power and disciplinary differentials and garner universal engagement of all team members. Procedural tasks such as the design of meetings, the establishment of standards for information exchange, and conflict management ensure constructive and productive decision-making, innovative problem-solving, and conflict resolution among team members.

Whitney et al. (2010) maintain that the leader's primary responsibility in any group is to help others to recognize their strengths and value to the organization through inquiry, inclusion, illumination, and inspiration. Inquiry addresses the aspect of ongoing dialogue regarding best practices and opportunities for positive growth. Inclusion addresses the aspect of creating a psychologically safe environment where all voices are welcomed and heard. Illumination is addressed through the use of appreciative practices, which highlight exemplary performance such as success stories shared via newsletters or at the opening of each team meeting. Inspiration is addressed by modeling leadership behaviors and by providing opportunities for positive change and

growth by 360-degree feedback in performance reviews and aligning job assignments with strengths and interests.

Much of the early literature addressed leadership with a capital L. It dealt with specific traits or situations that distinguished one person from the crowd, attracted followers, and inspired great accomplishments that were products of the leader's singular vision. Current literature conceptualizes leadership—with a lowercase *l*—as a constellation of behaviors that helps others recognize their strengths, articulate their ideas, and engage in collaboration with others in order to achieve optimum results. Although the leadership competency models described by Garman (2010) were formulated for healthcare administrators, the overarching themes of communication and self-management resonate for all members of the healthcare team no matter what their position in the system hierarchy. Put simply, self-management entails attention to process and people in the form of structuring the work environment and developing work relationships. High-level administrative turnover in the volatile healthcare industry highlights the importance of frontline healthcare workers assuming the leadership stance and becoming proactive in the creation and maintenance of resonant team cultures. Rather than *Leadership* being reserved for the few, *leadership behaviors* are viewed as requirements for all members of high-functioning healthcare teams. When leadership behaviors are the expected and respected norm of a group, traditional hierarchies break down, and active listening, knowledge sharing, collaborating, coaching, and continuous learning bridge the disciplines and enable the team members to achieve strong, sustainable relationships and provide exemplary patient-centered care (Becker-Reems & Garrett, 1998; Gittell, 2009; Institute of Medicine et al., 2001, 2003; World Health Organization, 2006; Spreitzer & Porath, 2012).

CASE STORY Finding Balance

Sometimes we get bogged down in the discussion phase rather than the decision phase. Too much input makes things more complicated and time consuming. We work very closely together and sometimes the social life of the team overtakes the more evidence-based work aspects. We call ourselves a "family." A discussion about a problem with a member can devolve into a gossip session. The whole conversation deteriorates and rather than using data and evidence, our feelings, beliefs, and concepts get interwoven, and we end up without a decision. We need to strike a balance between working with each other as a team and being a "family." What I do when this happens is refocus the team concentration. I say, "Hold it—Stop—Time out. That is fascinating, but here are the ideas on the table. What is the solution?" People appreciate the focusing.

—Karen J. Nichols, MD, Chief Medical Officer at Trinity Health PACE

REFLECTION: Leadership Development

"The longest journey of any person is the journey inward."

—Dag Hammarskjöld

Reflection is the process of changing one's perspective as new information and experiences are encountered. Leadership development is based, in part, on the ability to reflect on your own behavior and the effect it has on the behavior of others.

Think of a time that you assumed a leadership role in a group.

- Why do you think you assumed this role?
- What do you recall about your own behavior when you assumed this role?
- How did you feel when you assumed this role?
- How did others in the group respond to your assumption of this role?
- How did you know what they felt?
- What was the outcome?
- Did the outcome surprise you? Why or why not?
- What might you have done differently?

The Leaders as a Facilitator of Collaborative Space

Nundy (2021) describes the current and future landscape of healthcare as becoming "distributed, digitally enabled and decentralized." This means that care will continue to shift from institutions to patients' homes and communities. Electronic collaboration and virtual care delivery via phone and video will be more routine. Decisions regarding treatment will be in the hands of those closest to the point of care. As a result, the membership of health professional teams will often shift and will often be geographically distant from the patient and each other (Dinh et al., 2019; Schot, 2020; Tannenbaum et al., 2021). Team leaders and members will need to be mindful of the importance of relationships and communication in order to be interactively agile in unpredictable circumstances (Han et al., 2021). Edmondson (2019) suggests that leaders can build psychologically safe spaces by setting clear expectations and establishing a participatory environment oriented toward continuous learning.

Expertise—both in disciplinary specialization and teamwork expertise—is the team's most important resource. Interactive, teamwork skill, in tandem with clinical skills, are linked to positive healthcare outcomes. Teams perform best when the members are cognizant of each other's area and level of expertise. Knowing "who is good at what" is critical information in situations that require quick, coordinated decision-making. A clear understanding of the differentiation of individual knowledge and expertise among the team members facilitates the coordination of team action. It is particularly critical in more fluid teams since they must dive into problem-solving without the opportunity to develop teamwork expertise with that particular team (Burtscher et al., 2020). Effective coordination of expertise within teams dependson free-flowing communication. Leaders of stable or fluid teams bear the responsibility of creating psychologically safe spaces where all members feel free to "speak truth to power" without fear of retribution. Leadership that is affirmative, collaborative, and harmonizing has been linked with improved information sharing and question generation among team members (Zolno & Skillman, 2011; Hu et al., 2016).

Leaders and members of interprofessional healthcare teams can create collaborative spaces by mindful use of listening and questioning that stimulates discussion. Focused, productive discussion fosters engagement of all participants. Increased awareness of the range of disciplinary and team expertise within the group enables complex problem-solving in even the most challenging of face-to-face and virtual circumstances. Additionally, consciously compassionate conversations within healthcare teams have measurable effects in patient outcomes and employee satisfaction and retention (Brookfield & Preskill, 1999, 2005; Trzeciak et al., 2019) (**Table 6.2**).

Table 6.2 Questions That Stimulate Compassionate Conversations

Evidence	■ *How do you know that?* ■ *What data is that claim based on?*	Information seeking, not challenging
Clarification	■ *Can you put that another way?* ■ *What is a good example of what you are talking about?* ■ *Can you explain the term you just used?*	Give speakers a chance to expand on their ideas so they are more fully understood
Linking	■ *Is there any connection between what you've just said and what Alice was saying?* ■ *Does your idea challenge or support what we seem to be saying?*	Engage group members in leveraging each other's knowledge
Elaboration	■ *Why do you think that happened? How might that work here?* ■ *What are some indications that the plan may not be working?*	Promote problem-solving
Hypothetical	■ *How might that intervention have turned out if Mark hadn't voiced his concerns?*	Allow group members to use knowledge and expertise

(continues)

Table 6.2 Questions That Stimulate Compassionate Conversations   *(continued)*

Cause and Effect	■ *How might having our group affect our discussion?* ■ *What would including the patient in the discussion achieve?*	Facilitate critical thought
Summary and Synthesis	■ *What are the one or two most important ideas that emerged from this discussion?* ■ *What remains unresolved andcontentious about this topic?*	Foster application of new information and continuous learning

Data from Brookfield, S. D., & Preskill, S. (1999, 2005). Keeping discussion going through questioning, listening and responding. In *Discussion as a way of teaching: Tools and techniques for democratic classrooms* (2nd ed., pp. 101–123). John Wiley & Sons.

References

Anchor, S. (2012). Positive intelligence. *Harvard Business Review, 90*(1–2), 100–102.

Becker-Reems, E., & Garrett, D. (1998). *Testing the limits of teams: How to implement self-management in health care.* American Hospital Publishing.

Boyatzis, R., Smith, M., & Blaize, N. (2006). Developing sustainable leaders through coaching and compassion. *Academy of Management Learning & Education, 5*(1), 8–24.

Briskin, A., Erickson, S., Ott, J., & Callanan, T. (2009). *The power of collective wisdom and the trap of collective folly.* Berrett-Koehler.

Brookfield, S. D., & Preskill, S. (1999, 2005). Keeping discussion going through questioning, listening and responding. In *Discussion as a way of teaching: Tools and techniques for democratic classrooms* (2nd ed., pp. 101–123). John Wiley & Sons.

Burtscher, M. J., Nussbeck, F. W., Sevdalis, N., Gisin, S., & Manser, T. (2020). Coordination and communication in healthcare action teams: The role of expertise. *Swiss Journal of Psychology, 79*(3–4), 123–135. https://doi.org/10.1024/1421-0185/a00023

Dinh, J., Traylor, A., Kilcullen, M., Perez, J., Schweissing, E., Venkatesh, A., & Salas, E. (2020). Cross-Disciplinary Care: A systematic review on teamwork processes in health care. *Small Group Research, 51*(1), 125–166. doi: 10.1177/1046496419872002

Edmondson, A. (2019) *The Fearless Organization: Creating psychological safety in the workplace for learning, innovation and growth.* Hoboken, NJ: John Wiley & Sons.

French, R., Simpson, P., & Harvey, C. (2001, June). *Negative capability: The key to creative leadership.* Presented at the International Society for the Psychoanalytic Study of Organizations Symposia. Paris, France.

Garman, A. (2010). Leadership development in the interdisciplinary context. In B. Freshman, L. Rubino, & Y. Chassiakos (Eds.), *Collaboration across the disciplines in health care* (pp. 43–64). Jones and Bartlett Publishers.

Gittell, J. (2009). *High performance healthcare: Using the power of relationships to achieve quality, efficiency and resilience.* McGrawHill.

Gray, B. (2008). Enhancing transdisciplinary research through collaborative leadership. *American Journal of Preventive Medicine, 35*(2S), s124–s132.

Hammick, M., Freeth, D. S., Copperman, J., & Goodsman, D. (2009). *Being interprofessional.* Polity Press.

Han, J., Yoon, J., Choi, W., & Hong, G. (2021). The effects of shared leadership on team performance. *Leadership & Organization Development Journal, 42*(4), 593–605. https://doi.org/10.1108/LODJ-01-2020-0023

Holmes, J. (2015). *Nonsense: The power of not knowing.* Crown Publishers.

Hu, Y., Parker, S. H., Lipsitz, S. R., Arriaga, A. F., Peyre, S. E., Corso, K. A., Roth, E. M., Yule, S. J., & Greenberg, C. C. (2016). Surgeons' leadership styles and team behavior in the operating room. *Journal of the American College of Surgeons, 222*(1), 41–51. doi: 10.1016/j.jamcollsurg.2015.09.013

Institute of Medicine, Committee on Educating Public Health Professionals for the 21st Century; Gebbie, K., Rosenstock, L., & Hernandez, L. M. (Eds.). (2003). *Who will keep the public healthy? Educating public health professionals for the 21st century.* National Academies Press.

Institute of Medicine & Committee on Quality of Health Care in America. (2001). *Crossing the quality chasm: A new health system for the 21st century.* National Academies Press.

Institute of Medicine, Committee on the Health Professions Education Summit; Greiner, A. C., & Knebel, E. (Eds.). (2003). *Health professions education: A bridge to quality*. National Academies Press.

Klein, J. (2010). *Creating interdisciplinary campus cultures: A model for strength and sustainability*. Jossey-Bass.

Knowles, M., Holton, E., & Swanson, R. (2005). *The adult learner: The definitive classic in adult education and human resource development* (6th ed.). Elsevier.

Kolb, D. (1974). On management and the learning process. In D. Kolb, I. Rubin, & J. McIntyre (Eds.), *Organizational psychology: A book of readings* (pp. 27–42). Prentice Hall.

McKee, A., Tilin, F., & Mason, D. (2009). Coaching from the inside: Building an internal group of emotionally intelligent coaches. *International Coaching Psychology Review, 4*(1), 35–46.

Neill, M., Hayward, K. S., & Peterson, T. (2007). Students' perceptions of the interprofessional team in practice through the application of servant leadership principles. *Journal of Interprofessional Care, 21*(4), 425–432.

Nembhard, I., & Edmondson, A. (2006). Making it safe: The effects of leader inclusiveness and professional status on psychological safety and improvement efforts in health care teams. *Journal of Organizational Behavior, 27*, 941–966.

Nundy, S. (2021). *Care after COVID: What the pandemic revealed is broken in healthcare and how to reinvent it*. McGraw Hill.

Peterson, D., & Hicks, M. (1996). *Leader as coach: Strategies for coaching and developing others*. Personnel Decisions International.

Pew Health Professions Commission. (1998). *Recreating health professional practice for a new century: The fourth report of the Pew Health Professions Commission*. Pew Health Professions Commission.

Seppala, E. M., Hutcherson, C. A., Nguyen, D. T. H., Doty, J. R., & Gross, J. J. (2014). Loving-kindness meditation: A tool to improve healthcare provider compassion, resilience, and patient care. *Journal of Compassionate Healthcare*. DOI:10.1186/s40639-014-0005-9

Schot, E., Tummers, L., & Noordegraaf, M. (2020). Working on working together. A systematic review on how healthcare professionals contribute to interprofessional collaboration. *Journal of Interprofessional Care, 34*(3), 332–342, DOI: 10.1080/13561820.2019.1636007

Spreitzer, G., & Porath, C. (2012). Creating sustainable performance. *Harvard Business Review, 90*(1–2), 92–99.

Tannenbaum, S., Traylor, A., Thomas, E., & Salas, E. (2021). Managing teamwork in the face of pandemic: evidence-based tips *BMJ Quality & Safety*, 30, 59–63.

Trzeciak, S., & Mazzarelli, A. (2019). *Compassionomics: The revolutionary scientific evidence that caring makes a difference*. Studer Group Publishing.

Trezeciak, S., Roberts, B., & Mazzerelli, A. (2017). *Compassionomics: Hypothesis and experimental approach*. Cooper University Health care and Cooper Medical School of Rowan University.

Whitney, D., Trosten-Bloom, A., & Radu, K. (2010). *Appreciative leadership: Focus on what works to drive winning performance*. McGraw Hill.

World Health Organization. (2006). *The world health report 2006: Working together for health*. World Health Organization.

Zolno, S. (2007). Towards a healthy world: Meeting the challenges of the 21st century. *Linkages*, (34), 14.

Zolno, S., & Skillman, R. (2011). *Coaching certification in whole system IQ and appreciative inquiry*. The Leading Clinic.

© oxygen/Moment/Getty Images

Relationship-Centered Leadership Activities

Activity 1: Myers-Briggs —Your Leadership Behavior Under Stress and at Your Best

Using the following tables, write a profile regarding your leadership behaviors at your best and under stress. Think about a recent incident in a group where you were "at your best" and another where you were "under stress." How did you feel? How did the other group members respond? How can you use these insights to further develop your leadership skills?

ISTJ, ISFJ		ESTP, ESFP	
Dominant, Introverted Sensing		Dominant, Extroverted Sensing	
At one's best	Under stress	At one's best	Under stress
■ Are selective, choose the right facts ■ Have excellent recall ■ Are sure and certain ■ Reflect before acting ■ Communicate perspective to others	■ Fixate on the right facts ■ Obsess with minute data ■ Are dogmatic ■ Become paralyzed—take no action ■ Shut down	■ See and think, then do or say ■ Are active ■ Are talkative, sociable ■ Are straightforward and clear ■ Pay attention to detail	■ Speak and act without thinking ■ Are hyperactive ■ Chatter and disturb others ■ Are blunt and curt ■ Are pedantic

INTJ, INFJ		ENTP, ENFP	
Dominant, Introverted Intuition		Dominant, Extroverted Intuition	
At one's best	Under stress	At one's best	Under stress
■ Are problem-solvers ■ Are visionary ■ See connections ■ Make patterns ■ Have in-depth theory	■ Are arrogant, do not admit dependence on others ■ Have visions detached from reality ■ Are overly complex; everything is connected ■ Force data to fit ■ Will not ask for help	■ Form global pictures ■ Are innovative ■ Are enthusiastic ■ See possibilities ■ Are flexible ■ Are fast paced	■ Are obsessed with links between things ■ Are different just for the sake of novelty ■ Are frantic ■ Dither—cannot decide between too many options ■ Spin out of control
ISTP, INTP		ESTJ, ENTJ	
Dominant, Introverted Thinking		Dominant, Extroverted Thinking	
At one's best	Under stress	At one's best	Under stress
■ Persistently search for the truth ■ Have depth of concentration ■ Are logical ■ Are objective ■ Are self-motivated	■ Obsessively search for the truth ■ Are lost in concentration ■ Only his or her logic accepted ■ Become totally detached ■ Are driven—like a machine out of control	■ Are cool headed ■ Are rational ■ Possess clarity ■ Are logical ■ Are analytical	■ Are cold, detached ■ Think everything must be rational ■ Oversimplify for the sake of clarity ■ Insist upon logic ■ Dominate others by criticizing them
INFP, ISFP		ESFJ, ENFJ	
Dominant, Introverted Sensing		Dominant, Extroverted Sensing	
At one's best	Under stress	At one's best	Under stress
■ Are empathetic ■ Think people matter, including themselves ■ Are independent ■ Are sensitive ■ Are idealistic	■ Are rescuers ■ Carry the weight of the world on their shoulders ■ Isolate selves ■ Are hypersensitive ■ Are demagogic—thinking their ideals are the only ones	■ Are encouraging ■ Are interested in others ■ Seek harmony ■ Are outward looking ■ Are people and relationship oriented	■ Are insistent (e.g., "you will enjoy this") ■ Are intrusive ■ Ignore problems for surface harmony ■ Have a lack of focus ■ Are overburdened, overidentified with others

Data from Hirsh, S. (1996). *Work it out: Clues for solving people problems at work.* Nicholas Brealey Publishing.

Activity 2: Best Manager

Take a moment to think about the best and worst managers you have ever had throughout your working life. What adjectives would you use to describe your worst manager?

- Describe the specific behaviors this person demonstrated.
- What effect did this person have on you and others?

What adjectives would you use to describe your best manager?

- Describe the specific behaviors this person demonstrated.
- What effect did this person have on you and others?

Think about yourself as a leader. What three adjectives would you use to describe yourself as a leader?

- Describe your behavior when you are leading.
- How do you look and feel when you are leading?

Activity 3: Leadership Learning Journey

The leadership learning journey is a series of activities. Complete them in sequence. Begin with your lifeline and continue until you have a completed leadership learning plan. The leadership learning journey steps are the following:

- a. Lifeline
- b. Values Sort
- c. What Is Motivating My Values?
- d. Circle of Life
- e. Back From the Future
- f. Leadership Learning Plan

3a. Lifeline

Effective leaders reflect on all aspects of their lives. Reflective analysis of life experiences can assist in goal setting and charting a course for personal and professional development.

PURPOSE: To take a reflective journey to the past to explore in-depth impact, emotionally engaging experiences, and the lessons learned from those experiences.

Instructions

1. On a blank sheet of paper, draw a horizontal line.
2. On the left, write the year you were born. On the right, note today's date and finish the line with an arrow pointing to the future.
3. Along your lifeline, make a note of the following:
   - Important events in your life
   - Transition points
   - High moments
   - Low moments
   - Things you are proud of
   - Things you are sorry about
4. Include both personal and professional events and issues.

Be sure to pay attention to the emotions you feel as you fill in your lifeline. A sample lifeline is shown in **Figure PII.1**.

3b. Values Sort

Values are the foundation of who we are, what we do, how we feel about ourselves, our family and friends, our work or career, and how we interact with others. They affect our beliefs about what is right or wrong, and we often make decisions based on our values.

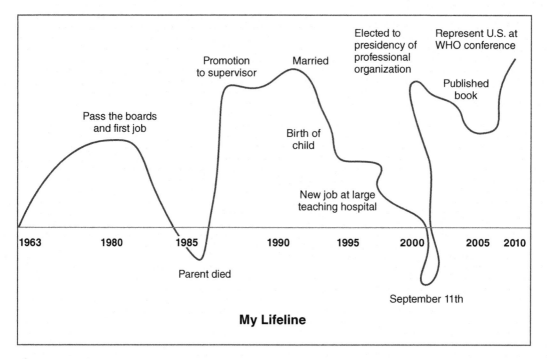

Figure PII.1 Example of a lifeline.

Instructions:

1. Look over the list of values provided. You can add to this list if your real values are not represented.
2. Select 15 values that are most important to you and mark them with an asterisk (*).
3. From the list of 15, identify the 10 values that are most important to you and mark them with a plus sign (+).
4. From the list of 10, identify the five values that are most important to you. Circle those five.
5. Rank your list of values 1 through 5, where 1 is the most important value and 5 is the least important.
6. Circle your top 10 values on **Table II.1** to see what motivates you to live by your values.

Values Sort List

Achievement
Accomplishment

Adventure
Affection
Altruism
Ambition
Beauty
Broad-mindedness
Calm
Challenging
Cheerful
Clean
Comfortable life
Competence
Competitiveness
Contribution
Cooperation
Courage
Creativity
Dependability
Discipline
Economic security
Empathy
Equality

Table II.1 Values Motivation

Motivation	Values		
Relationships	Affection Altruism Broad mindedness Cooperation Dependability Empathy	Equality Family happiness Forgiving Friendship Helpfulness Involvement Loving	Loyalty Mature love Peace (no conflict) Politeness Respect for life
Accomplishment	Achievement Accomplishment Adventure Ambition Challenge Competence	Competitiveness Economic security Fame Innovation Personal development	Recognition Risk taking Status Success
Influence	Contribution Courage Discipline Family security	Freedom National security Order Responsibility	Restraint Stability Wealth
Well-being, self-expression, and style	Beauty Calm Cheerful Clean Comfortable life Creativity Exciting life Happiness	Health Inner harmony Integrity Intellectual Logic Pleasure Power Religion	Salvation Self-control Self-respect Serenity Spirituality Wisdom

Data from Simon, S., Howe, L., & Kirschenbaum, H. (1995). *Values clarification*. Grand Central Publishing; McClelland, D. (1988). *Human motivation*. Cambridge University Press.

Exciting life	Loving
Fame	Loyalty
Family happiness	Mature love
Family security	National security
Forgiving	Order
Freedom	Peace (no conflict)
Friendship	Personal development
Happiness	Pleasure
Health	Politeness
Helpfulness	Power
Inner harmony	Recognition
Innovation	Religion
Integrity	Respect for life
Intellectual	Responsibility
Involvement	Restraint
Logic	Risk taking

Salvation
Self-control
Self-respect
Serenity
Spirituality
Stability
Status
Success
Wealth
Wisdom

Rank the five values most important to you (1 = most important, etc.).

1. _____
2. _____
3. _____
4. _____
5. _____

3c. What Is Motivating My Values?

Motivation is what incentivizes you toward action. When you are lying in bed in the morning, what inspires you to get up: getting something done (accomplishment), seeing your children (relationships), something else? Your values are often a product of your core motivation. Circle your top 10 values in Table II.1 to help you identify what motivates you.

Does this line up with your motivations? What else motivates you?

3d. Circles of Life

PURPOSE: To identify current state and future priorities.

We all have multiple competing priorities in our lives. Sometimes it is helpful to take stock of where we are spending our time and compare this to how we ideally would like to spend our time. For this exercise, list the categories of activities that are important to you. The list may look like the following:

- Exercise
- Work
- Spending time with my family
- Learning and education
- Spiritual practice
- Entertainment (e.g., movies, TV, social networking)

Now draw circles that represent the amount of time you spend in each area. Some will naturally intersect as shown in the following example:

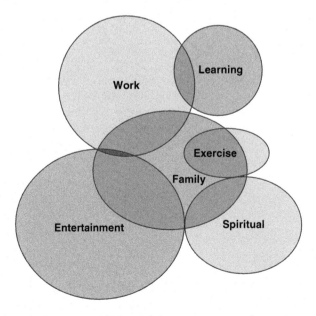

Category	Percentage of Time You Spend Now	Ideal Percentage of Time

If you like, fill in the percentages of the time you spend in these categories in the previous table. Add and delete categories for your Ideal column but be realistic (i.e., you probably do need to spend a good percentage of your time at work, but you may want to have your work overlap more with learning).

Now draw your ideal circles of life.

3e. Back from the Future

PURPOSE: Identify your ideal state of life 5–10 years from now.

Part 1: Fast forward to 10 years from today. Spend a few moments imagining what you hope your life will be like. Focus specifically on your role as a leader on an interprofessional team. Write a few words or sketch a picture of what your life will be like. You can include the type of person you hope to be, the people around you, the place you live, the type of leader you hope to be, your professional aspirations, and any other aspects of your life.

Part 2: Tell the story of how you got from where you are today to where you are 10 years from now. Start by filling in the blanks in the first sentence, which follows, and then continue with the rest of the story.

Today is _____ (today's date, month, and this year +10). I am now_____ (describe yourself 10 years from today). This is how I got here:

3f. Leadership Learning Plan

PURPOSE: To articulate vision, learning goals, milestones, and action steps.

Learning goals should be challenging and should include building on your strengths, as well as overcoming limitations as you develop these goals. Specific, measurable, actionable, realistic, and time-bounded (SMART) goals are as follows:

- *Specific:* A specific goal is better than a general one. Learning a new language is general. Learning Chinese is specific. Being a better leader is general; listening to team member input and feedback is more specific.
- *Measurable:* How will you measure your accomplishment? What will success look like? Examples include: I will complete the first three chapters of Chinese in *Rosetta Stone* in the next 6 months; I will articulate three messages (input/feedback) that I have heard from my colleagues each month.
- *Actionable:* Can you take action on this goal? Do you have the ability and resources you need to learn a new language? Are you approaching patient care from a client-centered and interdisciplinary way, and do team members give you input and feedback?
- *Realistic:* Are you willing and able to achieve this goal? Do you really have time to learn Chinese? Do you spend time with team members, and are you creating a safe environment for this type of communication?

- **T**ime *bounded:* What is your time frame for completing this? Examples might be: In one year, I will be able to hold a simple conversation in Chinese; and in 3 months, I will know enough about how members of my interdisciplinary team think to respond to the input with actions.

My Goals:

1. _____
2. _____
3. _____
4. _____

Leadership competency I need to develop: Continuously work to be a more strategic leader	
Action steps:	**Timeline:**
1. Read "Good to Great"	1. Finish by December 2012
2. Take a course in how to give feedback	2. January 2013
3. Create a coach who can help me: my boss; my colleague; my friend; my relative	3. By January 2013

Figure PII.2 Example of a leadership learning goal.

My New Leadership Learning Plan

Leadership Competency I Need to Develop (Goal No. 1):	
Action steps:	*Timeline:*
1.	1.
2.	2.
3.	3.

Leadership Competency I Need to Develop (Goal No. 2):	
Action steps:	*Timeline:*
1.	1.
2.	2.
3.	3.

Leadership Competency I Need to Develop (Goal No. 3):	
Action steps:	*Timeline:*
1.	1.
2.	2.
3.	3.

PART III

Building and Sustaining Collaborative Interprofessional Teams

"We prepare for an unknown future by creating strong and sustainable relationships . . . and by building resilient communities . . . human beings are caring, generous and want to be together. We have learned that whatever the problem, community is the answer."

— Margaret J. Wheatley, The Berkana Institute

CHAPTER 7

Leveraging Diversity Perspectives on Leadership

LEARNING OBJECTIVES

1. Differentiate surface-level and deep-level diversity.
2. Understand the concept of intersectionality.
3. Recognize and mitigate unconscious bias.
4. Apply communication strategies, such as deep listening, that recognize and respect the diversity of interprofessional healthcare teams.
5. Explain how inclusive leadership, cultural humility, and cultural competence foster innovative thought and creative problem-solving in diverse groups.
6. Manage conflict.
7. Create a psychologically safe team environment.

In the healthcare industry, diversity and inclusion are essential for providing high-quality care to patients from a range of backgrounds. Diversity refers to the differences that exist among individuals, including but not limited to race, ethnicity, gender, age, religion, gender identity, sexual orientation, and ability. Inclusion refers to the active and ongoing process of creating a work environment where all team members and their patients feel valued, respected, and supported. An inclusive, diverse team of healthcare professionals leverages the power of varied perspectives and experiences in order to provide care that is relevant to the patient population served. The amount and outward appearance of diversity varies organizationally, regionally, and internationally, and understanding its impact on teamwork poses challenges for leaders and members of interprofessional healthcare teams (Knippenberg & Schippers, 2007). Mannix and Neale (2005) suggest the following six broad diversity categories: social identity, knowledge and skills, values and beliefs, personality, organizational and community, and social network (**Table 7.1**).

Table 7.1 Mannix and Neale Diversity Categories

Category	Examples
Social identity	Gender, ethnicity, religious identity, sexual orientation
Knowledge and skills	Educational background, functional knowledge
Values and beliefs	Cultural background—family of origin, generation, personal history of experiences
Personality	Cognitive styles, temperament
Organizational and community	Status-like placement in organizational hierarchy, tenure, social–economic, respect for profession in society
Social network	Friends and work-related network of associates, family members

Data from Mannix, E. & Neale, M. A. (2005). What makes a difference? The promise and reality of diverse teams in organizations. *Psychological Science in the Public Interest, 6,* 31–55.

All of these aspects of diversity are salient to interprofessional healthcare teams and have been classified at the *surface level* or *deep level* (Harrison et al., 2002). Any dimension of social identity that has a history of intergroup prejudice, discrimination, or oppression (race, ethnicity, gender, religion, sexual orientation, nationality) is considered part of *surface-level* diversity even if it not immediately identifiable (Ely & Roberts, 2008). Deep-level diversity or psychological diversity is defined as personality, values, and attitude differences among team members (**Figure 7.1**). These are not immediately apparent but impact team function (Harrison et al., 2002).

Surface-Level Diversity

Surface-level diversity or demographic diversity can be defined as attributes that are physical, not easily changeable, and almost immediately observable. Age, race/ethnicity, and gender are all considered surface diversity. Social categories like organizational function, professional background, ethnicity, sexual orientation, and organizational status are also included as part of surface diversity even though they may not

be immediately recognizable. In those cases where demographic diversity is present but not immediately apparent, like ethnicity, religion, or sexual orientation, the term mid-level diversity may provide a more accurate classification. Most importantly, it is well established that these characteristics often form the basis for stereotypes—social classifications involving prescribed patterns of thought, attitudes, and behaviors (Fiske, 2000). Surface-level diversity has the potential to evoke a social identity threat through group stereotypes, microaggressions, and stigmatization (Steele et al., 2002). Threats to social identity can negatively impact team function resulting in social isolation, diminished communication, lack of attachment, reduced cohesion, and poor performance. Fortunately, it has also been shown that as teams work together longer, the increased opportunities for interaction around common goals tend to mitigate the negative effects of surface diversity (Harrison et al., 2002).

Deep-Level Diversity

Professional training and strength of professional identity often reinforce the personality, values, and attitudes that influence an individual's

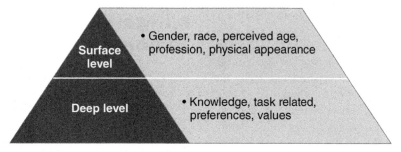

Figure 7.1 Dimensions of diversity: Surface and deep level.

choice of profession. Individual variation in these factors impact professional behavior. For example, a physician's primary responsibility is the health and well-being of the individual patient, while a senior administrator's primary responsibility is the economic viability of the entire hospital system. Both are legitimate and necessary orientations that may occasionally be sources of conflict. Not surprisingly, individuals prefer to interact with those who share a similar orientation because that interaction validates their commonly held beliefs, affect, and expressed behaviors (Swann et al., 1992).

Social identity theory suggests that people have a natural inclination to identify with and have an emotional attachment to others who are most like them in areas such as ethnicity, sex, race, and nationality (Hogg et al., 1995).

Intersectionality

Intersectionality is a theoretical construct that was developed to address the experiences of people who are subjected to multiple, overlapping forms of oppression based on their social identity. Specifically, it described how black women are subjected to a combination of gender and race-based discrimination and oppression that is compounded and different from the experiences of either black men or white women (Crenshaw, 1989, 2017). Over the years, the concept of intersectionality has been broadened to recognize the interconnected nature of myriad components of social

identity. Intersectionality views gender, ethnicity, religious identity, disability, and sexual orientation as overlapping and interdependent sources of discrimination, disadvantage, or privilege. An intersectional analysis considers the panoply of diversity factors that impacts an individual rather than considering each factor in isolation.

For instance, a gender and equity analysis conducted for the World Health Organization found that women are 70 percent of the global health workforce but hold only 25 percent of senior roles (World Health Organization, 2019). Other intersectional studies demonstrate how patriarchal advantage privileges white male nurses in leadership positions while studies done through the lens of professional orientation showed that nurses were underrepresented on health system governing boards (Aspinall et al., 2022).

While barriers to inclusion and leadership exist at the intersection of gender, race, ethnicity, professional cadre, and other socially constructed categories, so do tools for improving diversity, equity, and inclusion in healthcare teams. Some of these will be discussed in this chapter.

The Brain's Shortcuts and Unconscious Bias

In order for us to understand how to better work with diverse teams, we must understand the unconscious nature of bias. Unconscious bias, also known as *implicit bias*, refers to perceptions and reactions outside of our conscious control. These perceptions and reactions are triggered by our brain making quick judgments and assessments of people and situations.

The human brain is hardwired to quickly make sense of the world. In order to do this, the brain literally makes shortcuts in functioning that result in quick judgments and assumptions that enable us to take action or make decisions based on limited information and social cues. This survival mechanism enables quick physical reactions and cognitive efficiency when a person slams on the car brake to avoid an accident. As another example, you are reading this sentence and comprehending words quickly without reading every single letter in each word. These shortcuts are critical cognitive shortcuts, but they often work against us in human interactions. When we encounter another human being, we implicitly and automatically make judgments about that person, and our biases can blind us (Lieberman et al., 2014). Unconscious bias is largely responsible for assumptions we make about other people based on race, gender, age, facial expressions, and other subtle physical signs.

Recent neuropsychology research suggests that we have a prejudice network at work inside of our brains that includes the rapid processing of social cues in the amygdala (Amodio, 2014). The amygdala, a set of neurons in the brain, has emerged as a key region of study in bias research and is a focal point for understanding emotions. It is the part of the brain that reacts to fear and threat. Scientists have found a high correlation between amygdala activity and implicit racial bias (Ofan et al., 2014). Researchers have also noted that another part of the brain, the insula, is stimulated when encountering persons outside our primary social identity group and is related to a reduction of empathy (Bernhardt & Singer, 2012; Lamm et al., 2010). This tends to confirm that human beings have an easier time empathizing with those in identity groups that are similar to their own and less empathy for those who are perceived as different.

Mitigating Unconscious Bias

Interprofessional healthcare teams reflect a wide range of diversity including professional, racial, ethnic, and gender. Although more research to define the conceptual and operational parameters of unconscious bias is needed, it is clear that recognizing and welcoming diversity, in all its forms, is the first step in mitigating unconscious bias and facilitating more productive and participatory team functioning (Axt, 2017). Improving self-awareness and empathy and institutionalizing inclusionary practices are not only instrumental in mitigating unconscious bias in teams but are also associated with improvements in patient care and institutional financial performance. Gomez and Bernet (2019) found that healthcare team diversity is associated with reductions in clinical errors, improved patient outcomes, higher patient satisfaction, and improved revenue streams. Additionally, healthcare institutions that were perceived as having a commitment to diversity, in all of its forms, demonstrated lower levels of burnout and higher employee satisfaction and retention rates.

Research and experience support the efficacy of the following strategy for mitigating unconscious bias on teams:

1. **Accept** that the brain will default toward bias.
2. **Increase awareness** of biases by naming them (**Table 7.2**). Using self-report tools such as the Harvard Implicit Association Test can provide insight.
3. **Practice "allyship."** Create team norms that allow for safe participation and inclusion of all members. Actively notice, listen to, gather input from, and interact with team members who are underrepresented or marginalized (different disciplines, countries of origin, gender, race, age. etc.) (Luthra, 2022).
4. **Facilitate collaboration** by utilizing techniques like brainstorming, facilitation

Table 7.2 Naming Unconscious Bias

Social desirability	The tendency for respondents to answer questions in a way that looks favorable to others (most often applied to answering survey questions)	*Telling the leader what he/she wants to hear.*
In-group and Out-group	Favoring those you perceive as more similar to you over those who are less like you (in-group) and conversely perceiving those different from you more negatively than those similar to you (out-group)	*The physicians tend to dominate the meeting by talking to each other. The one member of color is rarely called upon, and the men's opinions are taken more seriously than the women's.*
Empathy gap	The tendency to underestimate the feelings of others	*Failure to take into account how a team member's job may be impacted by a change.*
Blind spot	Recognizing biases in others and not ones' own biases	*Talking about creating a more diverse team while hiring people who are all similar.*
Curse of knowledge	The more expert you are, the less likely you are to appreciate other points of view	*Making a decision and not asking for input.*
Availability bias	Making decisions based on the most accessible information	*Making a decision on treatment before getting all of the facts.*
Planning fallacy	Underestimating how long a task will take	*The team sets overly aggressive goals.*

rotation, and small-group discussion techniques like think-pair-share.

5. **Share planning and decision-making** by using tools like fishbone diagrams, force field analysis, responsibility assignment matrix (RACI), and design thinking.

Opportunities to Leverage Interprofessional Team Diversity

Teams that are homogeneous perform better in the early stages of a team's work life, while diverse teams—given the time to gain more information about each other and to work on group processes—are better at identifying problems and generating solutions. Ely and Roberts (2008) suggest that focusing on team goals such as improving patient care, creating better continuing-education structures, or implementing new technology is an effective strategy for channeling diverse perspectives.

Each individual has a personal worldview based on myriad social, psychological, and economic factors, and additional biases are imposed by professional or disciplinary culture. The lenses through which each member of a healthcare team views interprofessional teamwork may vary widely. For instance, every member of the team may have a differing view of who is considered part of the team. Is it the physician and the nurse? The physician, the nurse, and the therapy staff? What about the pharmacist and the health information manager? The dietitian? Are the clerical staff included? Transportation? A physician may view the team as governed by a hierarchy in which other members of the team are viewed as carrying out directives. Occupational therapists and physical therapists may see the roles between team members as more flexible and be more comfortable collaborating and negotiating disciplinary boundaries. Some mental health professionals may view themselves as autonomous and only engage other professionals as needed. What and how information is communicated is governed by each team member's perception of the team's composition, purpose, roles, and responsibilities.

The more closely aligned the members' perceptions, the higher the probability of optimum team performance and outcomes. At the heart of highly functional healthcare teams lies mutual respect born out of an interest in continually learning about each other, commitment to team goals, and making optimum functioning the norm. Reflection becomes the impetus and result of learning. Open communication, reflection, respect, and continuous learning facilitate the accumulation of social capital that sustains high-performance teams and organizations (Ghaye, 2005).

The need for a complex array of services such as medical, therapeutic, pharmaceutical, nutritional, social, and pastoral, as well as clerical, data management, transportation, infection control, medical supplies, and equipment management highlights the interdependence of all the stakeholders in the healthcare arena. For example, productivity in the occupational and physical therapy departments might be highly dependent on the efficiency of transportation services. Leaders and members who employ inclusionary practices such as soliciting input from all stakeholders in the healthcare process, recognizing successful practices, and consistently facilitating positive communication create psychological safety. Psychological safety encourages participation and engagement in collaborative healthcare practices. Mindful attention to relationship building mitigates the tensions that accompany interdependence. In the following case study, the physician was cognizant that her view of the patient might be incomplete and the transporter felt that his opinion was valuable and relevant to the successful patient outcome. As a result, the patient received safe and effective care.

High staff turnover presents a challenge for those who would attempt to develop strong healthcare teams. The culture of positive regard that is modeled by the leader and senior team members and adopted by all the members of the team creates a trusting and respectful work environment that transcends the behavior of particular individuals and facilitates the honest reflection and inquiry that is the bedrock of quality improvement in health care. By institutionalizing feedback strategies, power sharing becomes the responsibility of leaders as well as members who provide each other with constructive opinions and supportive advice. Meetings that are structured to facilitate universal contribution will demonstrate institutional valuation of collaboration. Senior team members who hold high-status positions or have been on the job longest have a unique opportunity to enculturate new team members by modeling relationship-building behaviors that facilitate interpersonal trust, respect, and active engagement in collaborator team efforts. A psychologically safe work environment is an important factor in staff retention and mitigates the risk associated with behaviors that bridge status differentials such as suggesting new procedures, offering unsolicited feedback, or sharing innovative ideas. The return on this investment in social capital is an engaged, loyal, stable workforce, and a vibrant, innovative work environment (Edmondson, 2019; Trzeciak & Mazzarelli, 2019). As the tenure of team members within a position increases, so does their communication and tendency to pay less attention to status differentials. As status barriers fade and team-wide collaboration increases, opportunities for creative problem-solving and innovation abound. The benefits

CASE STORY   **All Perspectives Matter**

A physician was preparing the discharge orders for a patient who would need help with dressing and transferring from bed to wheelchair. It was expected that she would be discharged to the care of her daughter. At the weekly meeting, the physician polled the members of the team asking that each person share any information they had about the patient. A member of the transportation staff *assigned to the rehabilitation unit had reported to the nurse that when he was transporting the patient to her final therapy session, she shared that her daughter had been injured in a car accident the previous day and she was in a neck brace. Further investigation by social services corroborated the report, and orders to discharge the patient to a skilled nursing facility were issued.*

of an experienced, competent, loyal, engaged, and stable workforce cannot be underestimated in any circumstances. In health care, the well-being of patients depends on it (Institute of Medicine et al., 2001, 2002, 2003). Time spent training leaders and members of interprofessional healthcare teams to be inclusive and to foster psychological safety is time well spent and should be incorporated into staff development initiatives for new and experienced staff (Nembhard & Edmondson, 2006).

Open Inquiry, Deep Listening, Inclusivity, and Creativity in Teams

Navigating the diversity of healthcare teams along with the complex and often ambiguous healthcare environment requires agile and creative problem-solvers. Health professions education places a premium on knowing highly specialized information. "Positive capability" in the form of skill development in areas such as clinical expertise and clinical decision-making are important competencies, but they are not enough to tackle the complex challenges of health care. The key to inclusive, creative healthcare team leadership is the combination of positive capability and the ability to approach complex or ambiguous situations free of preconceived notions (French et al., 2009).

Comfort with "not knowing" and the capability that predisposes one to be open to new ideas, or seeing things with new eyes was termed "negative capability" by the poet, John Keats, when he described the creative process of artists and poets (Holmes, 2015). This attitude can be expanded to include "cultural humility," which refers to the acknowledgment that we can never fully comprehend someone else's lived experience. At its heart, cultural humility requires self-reflection, awareness of our own biases, and a curiosity about our intersectional identity and that of others on our team. Recognition of the truly diverse nature of each member of the healthcare team, along with the recognition of personal biases, heightens cultural competence and the readiness to engage in conversations that provide new insight into how others experience the world (Luthra, 2022). Unfettered by the need to always have the answers, inclusive team leaders and members are poised to ask the right questions and actively listen to the myriad perspectives available within their teams (see **Figure 7.2**). Cultural humility, in combination with cultural competence, expands the healthcare team's cognitive flexibility, creative problem-solving, collective judgment, and engagement (Stanford, 2020; Khan, 2021; Luthra, 2022).

Health professionals who have cultural humility and a genuinely deep curiosity regarding diversity in all its forms can develop negative capability and become more adept at

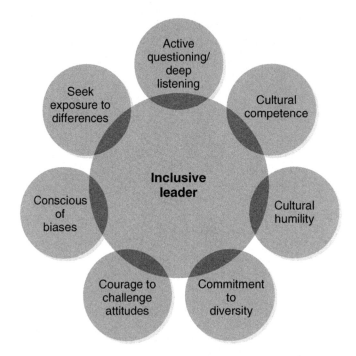

Figure 7.2 Inclusive leadership traits.

leveraging multiple perspectives in order to elicit innovative thought and creative solutions to complex problems (Hammick et al., 2009; Whitney et al., 2010; Khan, 2021). Knowing when to defer to the expertise of others is a valuable trait for leaders/members of interprofessional healthcare teams. The strength of the team lies in its ability to leverage the skills of multiple disciplines toward the common goal of client-centered care. While individual members of the interprofessional team have a comfort level with traditionally prescribed roles and responsibilities, they must be cognizant of the limits of their knowledge and capabilities and reach beyond disciplinary boundaries in order to facilitate relationships and client-centered versus disciplinary-centered practice.

By deep listening—refocusing our attention on the orientation of others—talking and asking questions rather than making statements, leaders/members of healthcare teams can transform disciplinary boundaries from spaces of conflict to spaces of new learning and innovation in relationship-based, patient-centered care (French et al., 2001; Gray, 2008; Klein, 2010; Stanford, 2020; Khan, 2021).

REFLECTION: A Different View
_____

- Choose an event (work meeting, speech, event from the evening news).
- Ask your colleagues to describe their interpretations of the event.
- How many different explanations did you hear?
- What did you hear that surprised you?
- How did it change your perspective?

Bridging the Gaps

It appears that the most effective leaders are those whose allegiance to group goals supersedes personal goals or who have a strong other orientation. Gray (2008) suggests that leadership behaviors in well-functioning interdisciplinary groups can be demonstrated through cognitive, structural, and procedural tasks. Cognitive tasks often take the form of appreciative forms of inquiry where the focus is placed on how the team can make best practice the norm rather than how the team can avoid mistakes. With specialized training comes greater natural resistance to alternative methods and approaches as well as greater difficulty communicating approaches to others who are not similarly trained. Bridging the gaps between the disciplines is often a key role that healthcare leaders play for their organization (Garman, 2010). Establishing strong social networks within the team and with stakeholders outside of the team are structural or bridge-building behaviors that serve to neutralize power and disciplinary differentials and garner universal engagement of all team members. Procedural tasks such as the design of meetings, the establishment of standards for information exchange, and conflict management ensure constructive and productive decision-making, innovative problem-solving, and conflict resolution among team members.

Managing Conflict

Health professionals often find themselves in positions that require negotiations with their peers, superiors, and subordinates. The discussions frequently focus on varied views regarding what constitutes best practice. Studer (2003) points out that proactive leaders negotiate with their constituencies in order to establish a set of agreed-upon objective criteria that represents a commonly held view of excellence. In the healthcare arena, objective measurements—whether they are patient satisfaction surveys, achievement of stated goals within a specific time frame, or a decrease in cost or increase in referrals—can serve as manifestations of best practice in action or excellent performance. Once objective criteria are in place, the team can focus on the key behaviors that contribute to excellent performance.

Fisher and Ury (1991) expand upon Studer's notion by noting that commonly agreed-upon objective criteria can help inform the development of a number of alternative solutions that are consistent with the interests of the other side. This demonstration of a willingness to be persuaded—of being open to new ideas—can engender similar attitudes in those whom you wish to persuade. A good negotiator assumes the role of problem-solver rather than adversary and is patient, flexible, and creative in the search for mutually beneficial solutions that are based on principles rather than positions.

REFLECTION: Listening with New Eyes

- Think of someone with whom you often disagree.
- Think of a topic in which both of you are interested.
- Ask him/her for an opinion/explanation on that topic. Sit quietly and listen to the answer without saying anything for a while.
- How might you encourage the person to just keep telling you about his/her perspective?
- What are the actual differences in your perspectives? What are the similarities?
- What surprised you?

CASE STORY Identifying Outcome Options

Many preschool children with special needs were referred to private programs for intensive early intervention, which included physical therapy, occupational therapy, and speech therapy. When these children reached school age, they received therapy services within their school systems. Parents who were accustomed to individual daily therapy sessions in the private settings lobbied for similar services within the school system. Teachers were concerned about the disruption that pulling children out for the various therapies might cause. The school-based therapists were doubtful that they could effectively manage such a large caseload, and the administrators had to deal with the restrictions of limited space, time, and financial resources.

All sides had the opportunity to share their legitimate, but sometimes opposing, concerns.

During the discussions, everyone was asked to express their main concerns. Not surprisingly, they shared a genuine desire to provide efficient and effective services for the children.

The commonly held desire for efficient and effective services was the point of departure for productive discussions about alternative, less-direct approaches to therapy that were more suited to the regular school schedule, such as program and case consultation, monitoring, technical assistance and in-service programming for teachers, and hands-on workshops for parents.

In the long term, many of the tools and techniques that were shared could be incorporated into daily home and school life—making both environments inherently therapeutic and effective in facilitating the children's development.

There is no doubt that this deliberate, strategic method of interaction requires time and skills, such as patience, self-regulation, empathy, listening, communicating, objectivity, and logic.

Questions tend to generate answers, while statements tend to generate resistance, so the successful negotiator should concentrate on asking good questions rather than making statements (Fisher & Ury, 1991). The more skillful one becomes in asking people for feedback and advice, the more successful one becomes in gathering the data that are most important to him or her. Focusing on another's felt need (not on personalities or emotions) helps to facilitate successful outcomes that contribute to excellent service delivery.

More often than not, successful patient outcomes depend on health professionals' ability to adjust their views to accommodate the views of others and negotiate many disciplinary perspectives. All perspectives are legitimate and meaningful to the progress of the patient.

Institutional excellence and effective leadership of interprofessional teams depend on the integration of various points of view. Communication tools such as team meetings, performance evaluations, productivity logs, and surveys are valuable means by which team members can share their perspectives and increase their effectiveness. It is within these day-to-day interactions that interprofessional curiosity, active listening, and principled negotiation techniques will afford the opportunity to engage in the ongoing process of establishing the most important things to the team. The consistent and reliable measurement of outcomes related to the important things will help all constituencies constantly assess their progress on the journey to excellence and provide clarification regarding if and when the definition of *the important things* needs to be reassessed. So, for example, a team may agree that it is important for soon-to-be discharged diabetic patients to receive training regarding wound care, but the administrator is concerned about financial and space restrictions, transportation services are concerned about getting patients to yet another location, and nurses and therapists have concerns about integrating specific techniques into the clients' daily schedules.

The common valuation of patient education serves as the point of departure for a discussion of all the possibilities, and the team agrees that a series of electronic training manuals, FAQ sites, or electronic discussion environments where questions, answers, and suggestions can be shared in an asynchronous manner might address all concerns as well as the most important thing in this case—patient education.

REFLECTION: Workplace Negotiation

Every day, we all engage in negotiations—big and small—in our workplace. Think of an issue that you and a colleague or colleagues disagree about. Take on the role of problem-solver rather than adversary.

- What is the issue that has to be negotiated?
- What are some of the interests that influence the positions of the people involved in the negotiation?
- What are some of the objective criteria that might be used to help guide the negotiation?
- List all of the outcome options for the noted issues/problems that are possible in your setting.
- How would you and your colleagues feel about the possible outcomes of this negotiation?

REFLECTION: What Is Most Important to the Team?

- How can you establish what is important from your institution's, supervisor's, or other team member's point of view? How will you go beyond your *assumptions* of what they think?
- How will this alter your perception of what the important things are?

CASE STORY	Interdisciplinary Teams, Building Bridges, and Culture Change: HIV/AIDS Intervention in Southern Africa

We worked with interdisciplinary teams that were involved in addressing various aspects of the HIV/AIDS crisis in southern Africa. These teams were made up of 100 individuals who were doctors, nurses, traditional healers, social workers, educators, United Nations relief workers, government officials, and media specialist communication professionals. Less than a decade before this meeting, many of these same people lived under apartheid, where roles and functions were strictly prescribed and biases ran deep. This diverse group of people needed to work together to reduce the spread of HIV/AIDS, deliver care to persons already infected with the disease, and distribute medicine over a vast geographic area where 30–40 percent of the population was affected by the epidemic.

The ultimate goal of this work was to shift the culture surrounding HIV/AIDS from stigma to respect and caring, from despair to hope, and from secrecy to self-disclosure. Workshops were designed to train the 100 team members as well as facilitators who could take the workshop design to others. Using experiential learning methods and appreciative inquiry techniques, participants conducted their own needs assessments and participated in focused sessions on emotional intelligence, gender, and age differences. They explored leadership, team dynamics, the causes and effects of stigma, and how to foster behavior change.

Through small- and large-group activities, people built trust and revealed personal life stories. Barriers among heritage, histories, and professions were crossed, and people found that they bonded across roles. Bonding as human beings went beyond the surface of teacher, doctor, nurse, social worker, and public policy maker. The establishment of collective goals and hope for the future transcended the pain of history. An appreciation for individual talents and the power of the collective evolved.

The collective energy that was unleashed by this experience spilled out into the community. Participants implemented their learning through projects such as a media campaign to encourage the use of antiretroviral drugs undertaken by a young organizer of an AIDS support group, nurses, educators,

and journalists. A compilation of videotaped interviews of southern Africans expressing their opinions of what they thought would help to rid the stigma of HIV/AIDS was created by a TV journalist, fundraiser, police officer, and social worker with funds secured from the Coca-Cola Company.

Every participant emerged from the training experience as a changed person—a change agent who continues to change the culture by transforming the lives and perspectives of others.

—Felice Tilin, President of GroupWorks Consulting, and Delores Mason, President of 2 Your WellBeing, Philadelphia, Pennsylvania

GUIDELINES FOR MANAGING DIVERSITY IN INTERPROFESSIONAL TEAMS

Moderate power dynamics.
- Make sure everyone has a voice.
- Start meetings with check-ins from all members.
- Rotate responsibility for leading meetings.

Focus on common professional values and goals.
- Create a common team identity. Take time to establish and articulate who the team is and what it stands for. Establish what is important to the team.
- Share variations in perspectives regarding commonly held values and goals.

Decide how decisions will be made.
- Decision-making depends on the task. Some tasks will require the expert to make the final decision. Some tasks may require consensus. Some will require a majority vote.

Create a safe, transparent environment.
- Establish ground rules for meetings and interactions and stick to them.
- Spend time getting to know each other beyond professional roles.
- Recognize the value of well-managed conflict.
- Seek the principle behind the position. Ask questions such as, "How did you arrive at that conclusion?"
- Do not defend your position. Ask for feedback. Making statements tends to generate resistance, while asking questions tends to generate answers.
- Recognize and reward success.
- Set up a time to articulate and celebrate team successes.

References

Amodio, D. M. (2014). The neuroscience of prejudice and stereotyping. *Nature Reviews Neuroscience*, 15(10), 670–682.

Aspinall, C., Jacobs, S., & Frey, R. (2022). Intersectionality and nursing leadership: An integrative review.

Journal of Clinical Nursing. https://doi.org/10.1111/jocn.16347

Axt, J. (2017). The best way to measure explicit racial attitudes is to ask about them. *Social Psychological and Personality Science*, 9(8).

Bernhardt, B. C., & Singer, T. (2012). The neural basis of empathy. *Neuroscience, 35*(1), 1.

Burgess, D., Van Ryn, M., Dovidio, J., & Saha, S. (2007). Reducing racial bias among health care providers: Lessons from social-cognitive psychology. *Journal of General Internal Medicine, 22*(6), 882–887.

Crenshaw, K. (1989). Demarginalising the intersection of race and sex: A black feminist critique of antidiscrimination doctrine, feminist theory and antiracist politics. *University of Chicago Legal Forum (1)*. https://chigacounbound.uchicago.edu/uclf/vol1

Crenshaw, K. (2017). *On intersectionality: Essential writings*. New Press. https://scholarship.law.columbia.edu/books/255

Edmondson, A. (2019). *The fearless organization: Creating psychological safety in the workplace for learning, innovation and growth*. John Wiley & Sons.

Ely, R. J., & Roberts, L. M. (2008). Shifting frames in team-diversity research: From difference to relationships. In *AP Brief, Diversity at work* (pp. 175–201). Cambridge University Press.

Fisher, R., & Ury, W. (1991). *Getting to yes: Negotiating agreement without giving in* (2nd ed.). Penguin Books.

Fiske, S. T. (2000). Interdependence and reduction of prejudice. In S. Oskamp (Ed.), *Reducing prejudice and discrimination* (pp. 115–135). Erlbaum.

French, R., Simpson, P., & Harvey, C. (2001, June). *Negative capability: The key to creative leadership*. Presented at the International Society for the Psychoanalytic Study of Organizations Symposia. Paris France.

French, R., Simpson, P., & Harvey, C. (2009). Negative capability: A contribution to the understanding of creative leadership. In B. Sievers, H. Bruning, J. De Gooijer, & L. Gould (Eds.), *Psychoanalytic studies of organizations: Contributions from the International Society for the Psychoanalytic Study of Organizations*. Karnac Books.

Garman, A. (2010). Leadership development in the interdisciplinary context. In B. Freshman, L. Rubino, & Y. Chassiakos (Eds.), *Collaboration across the disciplines in health care* (pp. 43–64). Jones and Bartlett Publishers.

Ghaye, T. (2005). *Developing the reflective healthcare team*. Blackwell Publishing.

Gomez, E., & Bernet, P. (2019). Diversity improves performance and outcomes. *Journal of the National Medical Association, 111*(4), 383–392.

Gray, B. (2008). Enhancing transdisciplinary research through collaborative leadership. *American Journal of Preventive Medicine, 35*(2S), s124–s132.

Hammick, M., Freeth, D. S., Copperman, J., & Goodsman, D. (2009). *Being interprofessional*. Polity Press.

Harrison, D., Price, K., Gavin, J., & Florey, K. (2002). Time, teams, and task performance: Changing effects of surface and deep level diversity on group functioning. *Academy of Management Journal, 45*(5), 1029–1045.

Hogg, M. A., Terry, D. J., & White, K. M. (1995). A tale of two theories: A critical comparison of identity theory with social identity theory. *Social Psychology Quarterly, 58*(4), 255–269. https://doi.org/10.2307/2787127

Holmes, J. (2015). *Nonsense: The power of not knowing*. Crown Publishers.

Institute of Medicine, Committee on Educating Public Health Professionals for the 21st Century; Gebbie, K., Rosenstock, L., & Hernandez, L. M. (Eds.). (2003a). *Who will keep the public healthy? Educating public health professionals for the 21st century*. National Academies Press.

Institute of Medicine, Committee on the Health Professions Education Summit; Greiner, A. C., & Knebel, E. (Eds.). (2003b). *Health professions education: A bridge to quality*. National Academies Press.

Institute of Medicine, Committee on Quality of Health Care in America. (2001). *Crossing the quality chasm: A new health system for the 21st century*. National Academies Press.

Khan, S. (2021). *Cultural humility vs. cultural competence—and why providers need both*. https://healthcity.bmc.org/policy-and-industry/cultural-humility-vs-cultural-competence-providers-need-both

Klein, J. (2010). *Creating interdisciplinary campus cultures: A model for strength and sustainability*. Jossey-Bass.

Knippenberg, D., & Schippers, M. (2007). Work group diversity. *Annual Review of Psychology, 58*, 515–541.

Lamm, C., Meltzoff, A. N., & Decety, J. (2010). How do we empathize with someone who is not like us? A functional magnetic resonance imaging study. *Journal of Cognitive Neuroscience, 22*(2), 362–376.

Lieberman, M., Rock, D., & Cox, C. (2014). Breaking bias. *NeuroLeadership Journal, 5*, 1–17.

Luthra, P. (2022). *7 Ways to practice active allyship*. https://hbr.org/2022/11/7-ways-to-practice-active-allyship#:~:text=Allyship%20is%20a%20lifelong%20process,the%20aim%20of%20advancing%20inclusion

Mannix, E., & Neale, M. A. (2005). What makes a difference? The promise and reality of diverse teams in organizations. *Psychological Science in the Public Interest, 6*, 31–55.

Nembhard, I., & Edmondson, A. (2006). Making it safe: The effects of leader inclusiveness and professional status on psychological safety and improvement efforts in health care teams. *Journal of Organizational Behavior, 27*, 941–966.

Ofan, R. H., Rubin, N., & Amodio, D. M. (2014). Situation-based social anxiety enhances the neural processing of faces: Evidence from an intergroup context. *Social Cognitive and Affective Neuroscience, 9*(8), 1055–1061.

Stanford, F. (2020). The importance of diversity and inclusion in the healthcare workforce. *Journal of the National Medical Association, 112*(3), 247–249.

Steele, C. M., Spencer, S. J., & Aronson, J. (2002). Contending with group image: The psychology of stereotype and social identity threat. In *Advances in experimental social psychology* (Vol. 34, pp. 379–440). Academic Press.

Studer, Q. (2003). *Hardwiring excellence: Purpose, worthwhile work, making a difference*. Fire Starter Publishing.

Sturmberg, J., & Martin, C. (2013). Complexity in health: An introduction. In J. Sturmberg & C. Martin (Eds.), *Handbook of systems and complexity in health* (pp. 1–17). Springer Science+Business Media.

Swann, W., Stein-Seroussi, A., & Giesler, B. (1992). Why people self-verify. *Journal of Personality and Social Psychology, 62*, 392–401.

Trzeciak, S., & Mazzarrelli, A. (2019). *Compassionomics: The revolutionary scientific evidence that caring makes a difference*. Studer Group.

World Health Organization. (2019). Delivered by women, led by men: a gender and equity analysis of the global health and social workforce. In *Human resources for health observer* (Issue 24). World Health Organisation. https://apps.who.int/iris/bitstream/han dle/10665/311322/9789241515467-eng.pdf

Whitney, D., Trosten-Bloom, A., & Radu, K. (2010). *Appreciative leadership: Focus on what works to drive winning performance*. McGraw Hill.

CHAPTER 8

Generative Practices for a Sustainable Collaborative Culture

LEARNING OBJECTIVES

1. Understand the importance of self-awareness, self-management, and personal renewal.
2. Recognize factors that contribute to resonance and dissonance in groups.
3. Utilize language strategically to foster collaboration, inclusiveness, and psychological safety in team environments.
4. Match dialogue and discussion to the developmental needs of the team.
5. Discover how strength-based and self-organizing strategies can facilitate positive organizational learning and change.

Professionals who are engaged in their work, committed to their personal and professional growth, share the organizational vision, and strive to accomplish objectives that have deep meaning to them are participants in generative learning. Generative practices are the techniques, methods, and support systems that foster generative learning and empower individuals to act as agents of positive change at all levels of complex systems (Senge, 2006). These practices facilitate self-awareness, self-management, communication, collaboration, role clarification, and reflection, which are essential interprofessional competencies (Interprofessional Education Collaborative Expert Panel, 2016). The key to the sustainability of social systems, like interprofessional healthcare teams and healthcare organizations, is the consistent attention to building social capital—those features that facilitate hope, vitality, self-efficacy, and relational coordination (Sampath et al., 2021; Treciak & Mazzarelli, 2019).

Only when we join ourselves vitally with others in arrangements of shared power can we reach a new threshold of co-creativity and purpose. This kind of empowerment emerges from individuals who are aware of and confident in what they uniquely bring to the organization and are focused on contributing their talents to create a healthier whole (Briskin et al., 2009, p. 90).

The following are practical methods by which individuals, groups, and organizations can foster a positive emotional climate, garner the infinite resources inherent to open systems, and enable them to adapt and thrive in an ever-changing world.

Individual Practices

Personal Renewal

In the high-stakes healthcare arena, health professionals are often at the mercy of rapid change, needing to take big risks and often making what may feel like life-and-death decisions for themselves and their organizations. This means that health professionals are likely to be in a state of high arousal much of the time. Healthcare professionals may be more likely to suffer from the burnout and compassion fatigue that is associated with taking care of others and not taking care of themselves. Ironically, sacrificing self-care actually reduces the quality of care provided (Landro, 2012; National Academies, 2019). This condition is magnified for leaders of healthcare teams who must navigate the myriad moral and financial challenges inherent to all healthcare organizations, who shoulder heavy responsibilities, and who are often distanced from people because of their position of power. It is not uncommon for leaders to succumb to the "sacrifice syndrome," which is described as a downward spiral of "internal disquiet, unrest, and distress" (Boyatzis & McKee, 2005, p. 6). Unmitigated entanglement in such a destructive cycle wreaks havoc not only on the individual leader, but on all of those with whom he or she comes in contact, resulting in poorly performing teams, high staff turnover, and poor outcomes (Hu et al., 2016).

In times of stress, the rational parts of the brain are likely to be affected by the more primitive, less rational parts of the brain. As physical and psychological capacity is overloaded, individuals are likely to react with fight-or-flight responses, and the overall capacity to be creative, solve problems, and learn is compromised (Alvarez-Buylla & Temple, 1998; Dickerson & Kemeny, 2004). While the sympathetic nervous system (SNS) is responsible for the body's ability to react quickly and effectively to physical or emotional provocation, the parasympathetic nervous system (PSNS) is responsible for recovery from such excitement and for keeping the body on an even keel by lowering blood pressure and strengthening the immune system (Goleman, 2003; McEwen, 1998; Sapolsky, 2004). As a result, a sense of well-being is restored and maintained (Diener & Lucas, 2000; Diener et al., 1999). A person who feels this way is likely to be optimistic, less anxious, and open to new learning and relationship building (Boyatzis & McKee, 2005; Frederickson, 2009).

REFLECTION: Daily Self-Sustaining Behaviors

The restorative nature of caring relationships, social networks, hope for the future, and mindful attention to the present stimulate PSNS activity and allow for intellectual, physical, and emotional renewal that is crucial to effective leadership and membership.

- What activities help you to feel energized and peaceful (walking, running, exercising, practicing yoga, meditating, painting, singing, dancing, or something else)? Could you see yourself starting or ending each day this way?
- What are the situations that make you most angry or anxious? Can you imagine reacting to them in a different way? Next time, before you react, ask yourself: "In this situation with these people, how could I move toward relationships?"
- How do you feel after you choose your reactions more mindfully or consciously? Are you more or less angry or anxious?
- What surprised you today at work? What did you learn? With regard to your work, what are you most grateful for? What do you hope to accomplish?

Self-Awareness and Self-Management

Self-awareness is an important prerequisite for self-management. Self-awareness is often facilitated through self-assessment, soliciting and using feedback, and a commitment to lifelong learning. Self-assessment tools include values, skills and interest inventories, and personality and type indicators such as the Myers-Briggs Type Indicator, Firo-B, and Kolb's Learning Styles. Self-assessment provides a direction for ongoing personal and professional development. Active engagement in self-assessment is particularly important for senior members of the healthcare team because subordinates are less likely to provide negative feedback (Evans et al., 2002). Goleman and company refer to this phenomenon as "CEO disease" (2002).

Multi-rater or 360-degree feedback instruments afford senior leaders an opportunity to receive structured, anonymous feedback from superiors, direct reports, and peers and are most effective when accompanied by coaching. Candid, constructive feedback alerts us to how we might leverage our strengths and bring about positive change. Consistent, focused solicitation of feedback from others demonstrates an investment in personal growth. The purpose of feedback can be appreciation, coaching, or evaluation. It is important to be aware of your attitude toward the particular type of feedback and the person or persons who provide it (Stone & Heen, 2015; Xirasagar et al., 2005; Crystal, 1994). Marshal Goldsmith recommends a feedback process he calls "feedforward." Since the past cannot be changed, feedforward focuses on how future actions can bring about positive change. Participants identify areas that need improvement and ask colleagues for feedback regarding what can be done to develop skill in this area. It is understood that the feedback is taken with gratitude and without any effort to explain or justify past behavior (Goldsmith & Reiter, 2007).

REFLECTION: Try Feedforward

Choose an area you would like to improve on. Choose two or three colleagues and tell them you would like to meet with them for a few minutes to do a "feedforward activity." In the meeting say to them, *"I am trying to improve on _____ in the future. Can you give me a few suggestions?"*

Write the suggestions down and thank your colleagues.

After you have collected all of the suggestions, read them and try implementing some of these suggestions.

Kolb's model of adult learning (1974) provides a guide as to how feedback can be utilized to foster lifelong learning and a continuous, self-directed approach to personal and professional development (**Figure 8.1**). After feedback is received, time is taken to reflect on reactions to the content and delivery of the feedback, identify a plan to address main issues, implement the plan, and reflect on the outcome.

Staying in Role

The ability to stay calm and focused on the goals of the patient, group, or organization rather than on personal needs and emotions is essential to every healthcare professional. Gordin and Trey (2011) refer to this as "staying in role" rather than "staying in person." Staying in person is an emotional, reactive state whereas staying in role allows for mindful attention to the task at hand. For example, a nurse who has just had a disagreement with a coworker but is able to focus and conduct a compassionate and thorough intake interview with a frightened and disoriented patient is operating "in role." On the other hand, if the same nurse was "staying in person," he might not be able to be empathetic because he let his emotions reign. Mindful attention to the goals of the situation interrupts the emotional messages from the amygdala, engages the neocortex or "inner leader," and facilitates an appropriate and effective response.

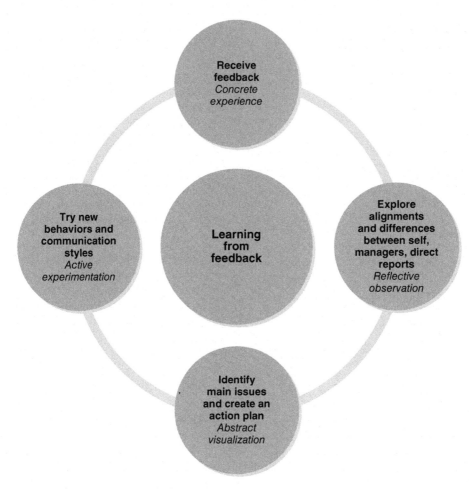

Figure 8.1 Kolb's model of adult learning.

REFLECTION: Staying in Person Versus Staying in Role

1. Choose a professional/work situation you have been in or will be in soon that is upsetting to you, and one where you believe your reaction to the situation may be out of proportion to the situation.
2. What would you do, say, and feel when you are "in person"?
3. Now, consider the same situation and focus on your professional goal in this situation. What would you do, say, and feel when you are "in role"?
4. Reflect on the differences. Did you say different things? Did you do different things? Did you feel differently?
5. Reflect on situations where you think being in role would be helpful to you and the outcome of the situation.

Interpersonal Practices

In order to navigate the complexity of our existence, we create mental categories that aid in the processing of experiences, feelings, and our perception of people. The cognitive organization or "chunking" of this data enables us to expand our knowledge base, plan actions, predict outcomes, and learn from our experiences. As new information is processed, emotional memories are intertwined with the lived experience. At each step along the neurologic pathways, our primitive brain in concert with our rational brain makes choices about what we believe we have seen, heard, and experienced (Dickerson & Kemeny, 2004). This cognitive process gives rise to the development of habits of thoughts and behavior that may be accurate, positive, and effective but may also be inaccurate, negative, and maladaptive (Langer & Imber, 1979). This is why "first impressions die hard." The research gives credence to this old adage and links emotions to in-the-moment behavior as well as to longer-term attitudes and judgments. For instance, we are often confused by, are mistrustful of, and have visceral reactions to persons who appear anxious, untrustworthy, or disrespectful. When we have experienced negative reactions to or from a person, we may develop a habitually defensive response to them rather than consciously choosing a response that is in tune with the current situation. We are likely to revert to mental and behavioral habits that may not be adapted to the situation at hand.

One of the manifestations of these behavioral habits is the tendency to interpret the behavior of others through the lens of our own habits of thought or personal bias. For example, team members might think, "Oh, of course Jim would see the issue only in terms of money. He's a finance guy." Or "Jane is always so resistant to anything new. We know what she will say so let's not even attempt to bring her in." Or "Mike always speaks first and thinks later." While there might be some truth to these shorthand observations, they are also stereotypical and may not describe the individual's current perspective.

In the absence of mindful attention to the perspective of others, misperceptions can often devolve into polarization and disengagement of group members. If group members feel that they are misunderstood and marginalized, they are likely to react in defensive and unproductive ways. Conversely, affirming interactions acknowledges the members' ability to move the group in a positive direction. They feel valued and accepted and will be invested in the work and the outcome of the group. In a resonant team, Jim would be valued for his ability to analyze the most cost-effective way to approach a project, Jane would be valued for her historical knowledge and ability to critically examine issues and identify obstacles, and Mike would be valued for his spontaneity, enthusiasm, and creativity. Hope allows for the consideration and valuation of all of the group members' strengths, dreams, and visions for the future. These acts of affirmation trigger a sense of wellbeing that sets into motion a positive contagion. The result is a resonant group that is calm, elated, optimistic, energized, and prepared to leverage its collective strengths and transform vision into reality (Trzeciak & Mazzarelli, 2019).

The following are some examples of how one might use affirmative language to handle a difficult situation by naming the behavior or issue that is of concern, acknowledging the negative feelings that it might engender, and redirecting those feelings toward a positive action.

REFLECTION: First Impressions

- What were some assumptions you made about team members when you first met them that changed once you got to know them better?
- How did this impact the way you interacted with that person?
- How did it enable or hinder the way you behaved on the team?
- How do you think quick assumptions facilitate or hinder the participation of individuals in teams?
- How do you think making quick assumptions might facilitate or hinder the output of the team?

Reframing

The affirmative language used in the following box is an example of reframing or the strategic use of language to highlight the current situation from a new perspective with the intention of broadening the repertoire of behavioral choices. The three sample statements in the next box are fatalistic, dead-end streets that lead the speaker and the listener nowhere. The reframed options provide a more optimistic and proactive view of the same situations and are focused on shared values, goal attainment, and action, and provide a variety of alternatives for action (Bandler & Grinder, 1975; Dilts, 1999; Hall & Bodenhammer, 2002).

EXAMPLES OF AFFIRMATIVE LANGUAGE

- We have every reason to be worried about this, but maybe we can brainstorm some possible strategies to head this issue off.
- We seem to have spent the last 10 minutes talking about Sally, and she is not even here. Maybe we can start to discuss how we can get this project done even if Sally cannot do what we think we want her to do.
- I think we all were disappointed that the last meeting with the patient didn't go the way we expected it to. I would like to discuss the lessons learned here so that we can do a better job next time. I know next time I will (provide bilingual instructions, make sure we are clear about team member responsibilities, engage the caregivers in the discussions, etc.).

REFRAMING EXAMPLES

1. Each health professional is trained differently. It is difficult to coordinate our intervention.
   Reframe: Having access to a variety of perspectives broadens the possibilities for innovative intervention strategies.
2. Finding a time when everyone can meet is too difficult.
   Reframe: Everyone's time is precious, and sharing information is crucial for good patient care. How can we use meeting time most effectively? When is the best time to meet? What are some other ways we can share information?
3. He didn't even respond when I gave my opinion; he just went on to the next person. It is obvious that he doesn't care about my opinion.
   Reframe: The meeting is almost over. It looks like he is trying to gather information from everyone while we are all together.

REFLECTION: Strategic Use of Language

We can use language strategically to facilitate a positive self-talk as well as positive team environment and stimulate positive action. Read the two sets of statements that follow. How do you feel after reading the first set of statements? How do you feel after reading the second set of statements?
Statement Set I:

- He is disrespectful of the contributions of others.
- I don't know why I took on the coordination of this project. It is too much for me to do.
- She is absolutely crazy! Ignore her.
- He is too pushy and tries to insinuate himself into things that don't concern him.

Statement Set II:

- He has a clear picture of what he thinks is best for the group. Could it be that he has a particular concern in mind that he has not shared with us?
- This is the kind of project that gets my creative juices flowing. I like doing the research and learning something new.
- Her view of reality is really vastly different than ours. We should discuss this further with her. Might there be a time/circumstance when her perspective could be instructive?
- He may seem pushy, but he really cares very deeply about them and wants to help in any way he can. Is his tendency to throw himself wholeheartedly into a task always a problem?

Group Practices

The emotional reality of a group, organization, or community is composed of subtle, yet powerful underlying emotional currents that affect the overall climate, culture, and behavior of the group. Humans react, on a neurophysiological level, to the verbal and nonverbal cues that we receive and transmit to each other and can generally sense when someone is upset or excited (Ekman, 1997; Gottman et al., 2001). This neural connectivity often facilitates emotional contagion—for good or ill—within groups. When a leader is perceived as angry, disrespectful, or unfair, these emotions are reciprocated and reverberate within the group, creating destructive emotional contagion or *dissonance* (Boyatzis & McKee, 2005; Goleman, 2003; Wang, 2022). *Resonance*, on the other hand, is synonymous with the positive emotional contagion that is generated in psychologically safe and inclusive environments (Ekman et al., 2003; Hatfield et al., 1993; Strazdins, 2000).

When routine interprofessional healthcare team meetings are characterized by positive interactive experiences, it is more likely that the teams will be able to respond in a rational, productive manner during times of stress. Conversations that are focused on the possibilities that each member offers for exemplary patient care are more likely to engage and sustain individuals, groups, and organizations and yield positive results in day-to-day as well as emergency situations (Ludema, 2001; Frederickson, 2003; Whitney et al., 2010). This concept is dramatically borne out by research on outcomes of emergency room team. Intensive care unit teams who viewed themselves as highly effective had lower morbidity rates, while teams who viewed themselves as more dysfunctional had higher morbidity rates (Wheelan et al., 2003).

Leaders and members of interprofessional healthcare teams can promote group development and team strength by creating and being attentive to opportunities for team interaction, discourse, and reflection. Closed-loop communication during routine interactions such as handoffs, debriefing, and huddling affords opportunities to clarify roles, responsibilities, and goals and share expertise and relevant information in a timely fashion. Closed-loop communication refers to the acknowledgment of the receipt of information and the clarification with the sender that the receiver has interpreted the information as the sender intended (Department of Defense and Agency for Research and Quality, 2014).

Something as simple as beginning each shift with reminders to be attentive to the situation (e.g., case volume), team performance (e.g., infection control procedures), and teammates (e.g., signs of fatigue) keeps the team engaged in mutual monitoring and attentive to the concerns of the team. Monitoring of the situation, team performance, and teammates along with consistent and comprehensive communication among team members will ensure that all the members have an accurate understanding of their domains of concern

Table 8.1 Shared Mental Models and Psychologically Safe Spaces

Personal/Team Focus	Situational Focus	Contextual Focus
How can you do that better? What skills can you use? What is holding you back? What do you need to know? Can you try it for a week? How can you contribute more? What support do you need? What are you willing to do differently? How do you suppose you could improve the situation? What are your challenges?	What is the opportunity here? What are the possible solutions? What is it we're not seeing? What is the challenge? What is another way? What if...?	What might be another perspective? How might someone else see this? Who cares about this? I am curious. Can you explain that to me/Can you speak more to that?

Pedersen, K. (n.d.). *Powerful question cards.* Growing Agile. https://www.growingagile.co.za/powerfulquestioncards/

REFLECTION: Responses to Nonverbal Clues

Our bodies respond to our emotions in subtle and obvious ways. Facial expressions, tone of voice, changes in skin tone, and postural stances may be fleeting but important signs of the emotions that drive a person's behavior (Ekman, 2004; Hamm et al., 2003).
   Think about a recent group experience you have had.

- Describe the nonverbal clues that you picked up from the people who were involved in the group interactions.
- What did the clues tell you?
- How did those clues affect your behavior?
- How did the clues affect the behavior of the other group members?

---

or a shared mental model (SMM). SMMs allow teams to develop "collective efficacy" and maintain resilience in the face of rapidly changing environments, high patient volume, high fatalities, and scarce resources. Some examples of questions that create SMMs and psychologically safe spaces for collaborative problem-solving are in **Table 8.1**.

   Appreciative attention to team successes and challenges encourages team members' willingness to take on leadership roles, ask questions, and approach problem-solving with open minds. In a psychologically safe environment, the team's shared perspective evolves along with the team's competence. In addition, using a growth versus fixed mindset to leverage opportunities for interaction and discourse can stimulate interprofessional collaboration. A fixed mindset limits the willingness to move out of one's disciplinary comfort zone, while a growth mindset welcomes the opportunity to try new ways of thinking and problem-solving (Dweck, 2006; Dinh et al., 2020; Tannenbaum et al., 2021; Salik & Paige, 2021). The following reflection provides examples of questions that can help to establish shared expectations, facilitate inclusivity, and orient the group toward continuous learning (Edmondson, 2019) (**Table 8.2**).

Table 8.2 Reflection

Reflection

1. At your next clinical handoff, debriefing, or huddle, use the following questions to establish a psychologically safe environment.
2. How did the interactions among the group members differ from other meetings you have attended or led?
3. How will this affect how you participate or lead groups in the future?

Describe Scope of Group Task	Invite Participation	Facilitate Growth
What are the goals of this group?	What are the ground rules regarding group member interaction and differences of opinion?	How can we model productive feedback?
What knowledge, skills, and attitudes are required to accomplish these goals?	Who are the members of the group, and what knowledge and skills do they bring?	How can we learn from each other?
What are the limitations of this group?	Who else needs to be included?	Are there other issues we need to consider?

The Team as Learner

McMurtry (2007) views healthcare teams as "complex collective learners with knowledge emerging at the level of the team that exceeds the sum total of individual team members' knowledge" (p. 38). The institutionalization of opportunities for interprofessional healthcare teams to interact on a regular basis provides fertile ground for the development of shared perspectives (Clarke, 2010). Strategies such as brainstorming and small group or pairs discussion facilitate inclusive communication and foster the development of a collective identity based on shared values, interests, and strong relationships. As a result, curiosity, hope, and energy fuel ongoing learning and build resiliency for all team members in the VUCA (volatile, uncertain, complex, ambiguous) healthcare environment (see Chapter 1). Interprofessional healthcare teams are often faced with complex problems. While the commonly held goal is the best possible patient outcome, diverse perspectives may often cause conflict. Psychological safety can make the difference between destructive and constructive conflict (Edmondson, 2019). Discourse that encourages team members to ask question,

express concerns, admit mistakes, and take risks contributes to the construction of shared meaning and a psychologically safe, inclusive environment within which highly competent teams thrive. The following approaches employ a team's communication capacity to establish a collective identity based on shared values, interests, and strong relationships. As a result, curiosity, hope, and energy fuel ongoing learning and build resiliency for all team members in the face of future change.

An interesting five-stage model for how a team might approach complex problem-solving is proposed by Wheatley (2005) (**Table 8.3**). The deliberate use of open-ended questions encourages behaviors and attitudes that foster discussion and collaboration and helps to create an SMM. Throughout the process, both leaders and members of teams can maintain a psychologically safe space by employing mindful, strategic, and inclusive communication.

In the training environment, simulation-based training (SBT) provides a natural space for fostering the interprofessional competencies of communication, collaboration, role clarification, and reflection through interaction and discourse. While SBT techniques

Table 8.3 Wheatley's Problem-Solving Model

Wheatley's Problem-Solving Model	
Stages	**Requisite Behaviors/Attitudes**
Cooling/Quieting	Patience/Curiosity
Enriching	Respect/Clear Thinking
Magnetizing	Generosity/Humility
Destroying	Discipline/Discernment
Acting	Cohesion/Reflectivity

Cooling/quieting: At this stage, each member of the team has an opportunity to share perspectives and understand how others perceive the problem. The following discussion questions might be appropriate for this stage:

■ What is the aspect of this situation that you think is most important?
■ What has been your experience in dealing with issues such as these?

Enriching: Differences of opinion are amplified and each side has an uninterrupted opportunity to provide a detailed rationale for its perspective. The result is a method for managing conflict and a more complete, collective understanding of all aspects of the issue.

■ What new learning did you experience?
■ How has your perspective changed?

Magnetizing: The broadened perspective provided by the previous stages help to foster a collective acceptance that there may not be only one best way, and the team may yet discover additional viewpoints.

■ Are we missing something?
■ Who else needs to be here?
■ What additional information do we need to have?

Destroying: Display a willingness to let go of things that are no longer efficient or effective. It is important to remember that any feedback is directed toward processes, not people.

■ Which things get in the way of solutions?
■ Which elements keep us from moving forward?

Acting: Employ deep listening and analytic skills to harness the collective wisdom of the team.

■ What is our intent?
■ How will we work together?
■ How will we support one another?
■ How will our work affect the patients, team, unit, and organization?

may vary in their focus, they all incorporate experiential reflection and debriefing. Debriefing is considered the most crucial element of SBT. Effective debriefing largely depends on the skill of the facilitator to create a psychologically safe learning environment and identify and bridge gaps in participants' clinical competencies and team dynamics (Salik & Paige, 2021; Klenke-Borgmann et al., 2022). In addition to the exploration and development of clinical skills, the sociological context within which these clinical skills are practiced must also be addressed in order for the simulation experience to be applicable to the real world. Prebriefing and debriefing sessions should explore how professional hierarchies, power relations, interprofessional conflict, and professional identity impact the clinical environment (Sharma et al., 2011) (**Table 8.4**).

TeamGAINS is an SBT model that fosters psychological safety and leader inclusiveness— important prerequisites for team effectiveness and patient safety. TeamGAINS encourages members of the team to broaden their perspectives and problem-solving efficacy by leveraging the knowledge, skills, and attitudes of their teammates. Additionally, any training method must take into account the need to prepare health professionals to be members of "action teams": *"teams of highly skilled specialists who work together for brief performance events requiring flexibility, and improvisation in an unpredictable context, often under high time pressure and with unstable team membership. Rather than functioning via long-term planning or team building action teams rely on adaptive coordination during brief performance sequences"* (Kolbe, et al., 2013).

Table 8.4 Sample: A Simulation Debriefing for Interprofessional Education

Simulations can take many forms in face-to-face or virtual environments. Simulations routinely include pretest, briefing, scenario running, and debriefing (International Nursing Association of Clinical and Simulation Learning, 2021). This example focuses on debriefing and consists of setting the scene, reactions, description, analysis, and application/summary (Chen et al., 2016). Sample phrases show how a facilitator might use language to highlight teamwork and collaboration.

Setting the Scene

Objective: Create a safe context for learning.

Facilitator task: Articulate the basic assumptions.

Sample phrases: *"You have reviewed the video. Let's spend 30 minutes debriefing."*
"Our goal is to improve how we work together as a team and care for this patient."
"Everyone here wants to improve."

Reactions

Objective: Explore feelings.

Facilitator task: Solicit initial reactions.

Sample phrases: *"How are you feeling?"*
"Any initial reactions?"
"What clinical challenges did you confront?"
"How did they affect your teamwork?"

Description

Objective: Develop a shared understanding of the case.

Facilitator task: Establish the disciplinary perspective of each team member.

Sample phrases: *"What were the key issues in this case?"*
"What special interventions did this patient require?"
"How did your professional expertise impact the clinical decision-making in this case?"

Analysis

Objective: Identify discipline-specific clinical competencies as well as interprofessional competencies.

Facilitator task: Focus on communication, collaboration, and role clarification.

(continues)

Table 8.4 Sample: A Simulation Debriefing for Interprofessional Education   *(continued)*

Sample phrases: *"I'd like to spend some time on your individual performance because each of your professions has distinct expectations."*
"Your ability to demonstrate these competencies make each of your contributions to the team unique."
"How did you leverage each other's expertise?"
"How were decisions made?"
"Did you perceive any power differentials?"
"Was there any evidence of conflict?"
"How was conflict resolved?"

Application/Summary

Objective: Identify common takeaways.

Facilitator task: Focus on both student-centered and team-centered takeaways.

Sample Phrases: *"What are some takeaways from the discussion for your individual professional development and our common clinical practice in acute care?"*

Organizational Practices

Complex systems such as healthcare organizations require problem-solving and organizational change strategies that consider diverse, often opposing perspectives from a broad range of stakeholders. A continuously learning system is a psychologically safe system where management and information technology practices are intentionally designed to support and stimulate asking questions, expressing concerns, admitting mistakes, and proposing innovative ways to solve problems (Sampath et al., 2021; Edmondson, 2019; Goodwin, 2017).

While standardization of communication tools, like checklists, assessments, care planning, and handoff protocols, and tiered huddles provide consistent and valuable opportunities to create a collective reality and provide for collaborative discourse, their effectiveness and acceptance by teams depends on team competence. Likewise, information and communication technologies may provide new and effective tools to promote collaboration, but their effectiveness will always depend on the organizational ethos and the nature of the interprofessional relationships with the organization (Goodwin, 2017). This means that leaders and members of teams need to remain vigilant and attentive to social–psychological aspects of teams (Eppich et al., 2016).

Schot et al. (2020) describe categories for interprofessional collaboration: bridging gaps, negotiating overlaps, and creating spaces. Sharing differing professional perspectives is an example of bridging gaps. Clarifying work roles and responsibilities is an example of negotiating overlaps. Creating spaces refers to arrangements for meeting time, place, and virtual or face-to-face interaction. Much of the collaboration in hospital settings appear to be in the category of bridging gaps, while negotiating behaviors characterized collaboration in primary and neighborhood care. No matter where teams practice, whether or not they are professionally diverse or face to face or virtual, the literature shows that a psychologically safe environment is linked to optimum performance (Edmondson, 2019; Trezebiak, & Mazzerrelli, 2019).

Tiered, escalating daily huddles are an example of how to ensure that each level of the organization has an opportunity to share information and provide feedback regarding care for patients, caregivers, and the organization. Each day, meetings occur, sequentially, at every level of care—unit, department, and executive. Information from all clinical and administrative levels is moved up and down the chain of command so that successes, problems, resolutions, and learning are shared throughout the organization. The institutionalized commitment to the consistent flow of information fosters the interprofessional competencies of communication, collaboration, role clarification, and reflection and creates a culture of continuous learning throughout the organization (Sampath et al., 2021).

Research has emphasized how managers, educators, and policy makers can institutionalize interprofessional collaboration (Atwal & Caldwell, 2002; Valentijn et al., 2013). However, in the current context of health care, which is increasingly more distributed, digitally enabled, and decentralized, the key to sustaining a collaborative culture is a commitment by all stakeholders to an inclusive, psychologically safe environment (Nundy, 2021; Schot et al., 2020; Edmondson, 2019). The following approaches encourage members at all system levels to actively engage in the process of analyzing complex problems and designing multifaceted, sustainable solutions.

Appreciative Inquiry

Appreciative inquiry (AI) is an approach to personal and organizational change that is rooted in positive psychology and based on the belief that the study of what is positive about individuals and systems will help to create positive images and actions in those systems (Cooperrider et al., 2008). AI leverages the power of diversity in groups and the infinite relational capacity of human social systems. The energy created by positive inquiry and dialogue generates productive individual and collective action and sustainable success. AI approaches are uniquely suited to interprofessional healthcare teams because their inherent diversity provides opportunities for fruitful conversations, infinite relational possibilities, and innovative action plans.

The practice of AI has conceptual roots in positive psychology and social constructivist theory and is informed by eight essential principles regarding human organizing and change:

1. The **constructionist principle** recognizes the centrality of communication and language to the change process and that reality is an interactive, dialogic construct. The constructionist principle posits that words create worlds.
2. The **simultaneity principle** suggests that change begins at the moment of inquiry.
3. The **poetic principle** suggests that the metaphors and narratives that groups develop can influence the outcome of their collective action.
4. The **anticipatory principle** maintains that positive and hopeful images of the future engender a positive approach to present circumstances.
5. The **positive principle** proposes that affirmative questions elicit positive affect, which, in turn, provides the energy and engagement required for positive change and growth.
6. The **wholeness principle** states that engaging all stakeholders in a process increases creative alternatives for action and ensures collective investment and engagement.
7. The **enactment principle** claims "positive change occurs when the process used to create the change is a living model of the ideal future" (Whitney et al., 2010, p. 52).
8. The **free-choice principle** suggests that performance improves when individuals are free to work in a manner consistent with their talents and values.

REFLECTION: Personal Appreciative Inquiry

- Describe a high point in your career as a health professional.
- What particular personal qualities of yours made this possible?
- What is the aspect of your work that makes it most engaging and meaningful for you?
- If you had three wishes for making your work even more engaging and meaningful, what would they be?

Simply stated, AI is an open, system-wide dialogic approach that focuses on the study of the positive core of an individual, group, or organization. An AI initiative can span from two to three hours to more extended periods of time, depending on the needs of the team or organization. The inclusive nature of AI affords each participant an active voice and an opportunity to dream together and experience their contributions as instrumental in the ongoing creation of a collective vision for the future. The AI process is conceptualized as a four-stage cycle that includes discovery, dream, design, and destiny. This cycle powers the direction for the inquiry and builds a positive foundation upon which human systems can grow and change.

The process begins with the team or organization establishing the topics that they wish to study. Healthcare teams might begin with questions such as: What does this healthcare organization look like when it is at its best? How can the best become the norm? Appropriate AI topics are stated in the affirmative and represent areas about which all constituencies are curious and interested in developing. Topics in healthcare venues might be improving patient care, establishing a relationship-centered organization, fostering wellness behaviors in patients and staff, and increasing the effectiveness of interprofessional teams.

The discovery stage helps participants reflect on their positive core and employs interviewing as broad a constituency as possible in order to elucidate the perceived strengths and potentials of the whole team or organization. Interview questions at this stage fall into three broad categories that focus on the past, the present, and the future.

During the dream stage, the group is invited to imagine how the best performance can become better. The group uses its collective hope to create positive imagery for the future. Based on the anticipatory principle, it is expected that groups will gravitate toward their co-constructed image of the future. In other words, if the group's self-talk is positive, the likelihood of positive outcomes will be increased. It is crucial that a wide assortment of perspectives inform this dream of the future. There are a variety of ways to unleash the full potential of a group's or organization's imagined future. Whitney et al. (2010) provide an example of how a company that managed several long-term care facilities used the dream stage of an appreciative inquiry to create a foundation for a strategic business plan while strengthening a team culture. The group was asked to imagine the world 10 and 20 years into the future when they, personally, were in need of an extended care facility. The group was then asked to address the following questions: What are some of the positive trends in the industry that give you the

---

STAGE 1: Discovery

Appreciative Interview Question (Example)

- Describe successful interprofessional teams in which you were a member/leader.
- Describe a high point of the team. What did it feel like?
- What did you do to make the team successful?
- What did the members do?
- What individual, group, and organizational resources contribute to the success of the team?
- What are your hopes for this team?

greatest hope for the future of long-term care? Based on those trends, identify six strategic business opportunities that might emerge in the next 10 years. The answers to those questions served as the basis for design and destiny phases of the AI cycle.

The design stage enables the group to influence its destiny by choosing the opportunities that are most congruent with their collective values and beliefs. The group begins to focus on those aspects of the social architecture—or organizational design elements—that will be targeted. Some components of an interprofessional social architecture would be vision, purpose, leadership, decision-making, communication systems, roles, services, policies, and procedures. One of the key decisions in the design phase is the creation of a positive description of the ideal organization along with propositions regarding how the ideal will be realized. These

propositions are stated in the present tense—as if they already exist; they are based on narratives of best practice that were shared in the discovery phase. They transcend current practice and are linked to the aspirations of the group.

The destiny phase allows the participants to establish how they will celebrate their accomplishments and initiate goal-driven action plans and methods for systematically assessing progress. The action plans are informed by the provocative propositions developed in Stage 3. Stage 4 has the following key questions: What are the changes that have occurred as a result of our inquiry? How will we communicate and celebrate the progress we have made? How will we recognize and reward exemplary performance and innovation? What are the time, resources, and personnel needed to support the planned actions, programs, or processes?

STAGE 2: Dream

Future Focus Question (Example)
   Imagine 10 years into the future.
- What are some of the positive trends in health care that give you the greatest hope for the future of the services that your team provides (e.g., adult rehabilitation services, wellness education, school-based pediatric services)?
- Based on those trends, identify six strategic opportunities for improving patient/client outcomes that might emerge in the next 5 years.

STAGE 3: Design

Provocative Proposition (Example)
   Design Element: Communication
   Open and honest communication among all members of the team is essential for efficient and effective healthcare services. All members of the team trust that their input is valued and important and recognize that their active participation is necessary for optimum patient care and outcomes. Meetings are structured to ensure that every member of the team has a voice. Decision-making processes are patient centered and relationship centered.

STAGE 4: Destiny

Celebrate, Generate, Collaborate for Action (Example)
During your interviews, you heard many stories regarding what makes a successful team.

- What were some examples of situations where all members of the team participated in open and honest communication? How were decisions made?
- Since we have begun this inquiry, what are some of the positive changes that you have noticed in your team?
- What management practices, human resource programs, or work processes would help to make inclusive communication the norm in your team?
- What are the time, resources, and personnel that would be required to support and institutionalize these practices?
- How will you recognize exemplary performance and progress?

Open Space Technology

This open, self-organized, and participant-driven meeting design has its roots in complexity science, which recognizes that patterns or order emerge naturally in complex adaptive systems as a result of the interaction of the systems' parts. Open space is appropriate in any situation that is marked by urgent, conflict-prone, complex issues that need to be addressed by many perspectives. Since all participants contribute to the creation of agenda topics and ultimately identify focal issues and action plans, it is expected that they will be committed to the implementation of those plans. The four basic principles and one law that govern open space technology reflect that the responsibility for the learning and outcomes of the meeting rests with each individual participant (Peterson, 2009; Owen, 2008).

1. *Whoever comes are the right people.* Since each individual has the opportunity to define the agenda and choose which discussions to participate in, it is assumed that they are committed to the issue and doing something about it.
2. *Whatever happens is the only thing that could have happened.* This implies that the focus is on the present with the people who are present.
3. *Whenever it starts is the right time.* Do the best you can within the allotted time frame.
4. *When it's over, it's over.* Then move on.
5. *The law of two feet.* If you find yourself neither learning nor contributing, use your two feet to move to a discussion where you are learning/contributing.

Examples of Open Space Initiatives

A large number of hospital and family practice physicians meet with hospital administration in an Open Space forum and create over 20 proposals for clinical innovations. The group analyzes the proposals and is able to establish priorities and a time line for implementation.

An Open Space initiative is used to coordinate regional healthcare services. Events made up of 300-500 stakeholders explore viable health services options and priorities. Priorities are provided to regional boards of health and form the basis for the coordination of cross regional healthcare services.

Data from Peterson, L. (2009, July 25). Healthcare and open space technology. Retrieved from http://www.plexusinstitute.org/resource/collection /6528ED29-9907-4BC7-8D00-8DC907679FED/open_space_and_healthcare_larry_peterson_article_8-09.doc

World Café Approach

The World Café Approach (World Café, 2015) is a form of nominal group process or structured brainstorming designed to facilitate the production of knowledge and action. The purpose of the World Café is to foster collaboration, group engagement, idea generation, and decision-making. This inclusive approach allows people of diverse perspectives to be collaborators who explore questions that matter to them, identify new insights, and develop the cognitive flexibility that is required for creative solutions to complex problems.

The need for self-actualization and to connect with others is central to the evolutionary process of human systems. Teams gain and sustain vitality when leaders and members can find balance between individual and collective needs and focus on a common vision and goals. Consistent positive interactions mitigate workplace stress, facilitate personal renewal, and lay the groundwork for an affirmative, hopeful, team-oriented culture. Ever-expanding relational networks increase the self-efficacy of leaders and members and facilitate group development. As teams mature, leadership and responsibility for outcomes become more evenly assumed. The resultant increase in leader and member self-efficacy renders the team more resilient, adaptive, and successful—all of which contribute to the team's overall sustainability. There is no one way for leaders and members to make interprofessional healthcare teams sustainable in the face of change. The path to sustainability of cultures, organizations, and teams seems less related to the answers we think we have than the questions we are brave enough to ask. How can we leverage our diverse perspectives? How can we maintain a patient- and relationship-centered practice? How can we increase the number, variety, and strength of connections? It is this ongoing process of inquiry that will keep leaders and members of interprofessional healthcare teams operating strategically and effectively in facilitating positive change and growth in themselves and in those whom they aspire to serve.

Example of A World Café

The Sunrise Health System needs to establish a focus on community engagement. Administration, clinicians, staff, and community representatives have been gathered together for a World Café. They will explore the following questions:

- What are your personal values and how do they relate to your work at Sunrise Health System?
- What does the concept of community mean to you and how might it relate to the community we serve?
- In what ways might Sunrise Health System serve our broadly defined community?

Three tables have been set up. Each table will focus on one of the questions. There will be three discussion rounds, each lasting about 20 minutes. At the end of each round, participants will move to the next table. As participants begin the next round, the table host will welcome travelers from other tables for the upcoming round, share key insights from the previous round, and encourage the jotting down of connections, patterns, and deeper questions. At the end of the three rounds, question headings will be posted and all the ideas will be harvested by having participants post ideas gleaned from discussions under the relevant question headings. The whole group will convene and identify patterns, themes, insights, action plans, and new questions. The collaborative community may be broadened and sustained by establishing online discussion forums.

References

Alvarez-Buylla, A., & Temple, S. (1998). Stem cells in the developing and adult nervous system. *Journal of Neurobiology, 36*(2), 105–110.

Bandler, R., & Grinder, J. (1975). *The structure of magic, volume II: A book about communication and change.* Science and Behavior Books.

Boyatzis, R., & McKee, A. (2005). *Resonant leadership.* Harvard Business School Press.

Briskin, A., Erickson, S., Ott, J., & Callanan, T. (2009). *The power of collective wisdom and the trap of collective folly.* Berrett-Koehler.

Cheng, A., Grant, V., Robinson, T., Catena, H., Lachapelle, K., Kim, J., ... & Eppich, W. (2016). The Promoting Excellence and Reflective Learning in Simulation (PEARLS) approach to health care debriefing: a faculty development guide. *Clinical Simulation in Nursing, 12*(10), 419–428.

Clarke, D. (2010). Achieving teamwork in stroke units: The contribution of opportunistic dialogue. *Journal of Interprofessional Care, 24*(3), 285–297.

Cooperrider, D., Whitney, D., & Stavros, J. (2008). *Appreciative inquiry handbook: For leaders of change.* Crown Custom Publishing.

Crystal, B. (1994). The 360 degree assessment. *Healthcare Executive, 9*(6), 18–21.

Department of Defense and Agency for Research and Quality. (2014). *TeamsSTEPPS fundamentals course: Module 3. Communication.* https://www.ahrq.gov/teamstepps/instructor/fundamentals/module3/igcommunication.html

Dickerson, S., & Kemeny, M. (2004). Acute stressors and cortisol responses: A theoretical integration and synthesis of laboratory research. *Psychological Bulletin, 130*, 355–391.

Diener, E., & Lucas, R. (2000). Subjective emotional well-being. In M. Lewis & J. Haviland-Jones (Eds.), *Handbook of emotion* (2nd ed., pp. 325–337). Guilford.

Diener, E., Suh, E., Lucas, R., & Smith, H. (1999). Subjective well-being: Three decades of progress. *Psychological Bulletin, 125*, 276–302.

Dilts, R. (1999). *Sleight of mouth: The magic of conversational belief change.* Meta Publishers.

Dinh, J. V., Traylor, A. M., Kilcullen, M. P., Perez, J. A., Schweissing, E. J., Venkatesh, A., & Salas, E. (2020). Cross-disciplinary care: A systematic review on team work processes in health care. *Small Group Research, 51*(1), 125–166. doi:10.1177/1046496419872002

Dweck, C. S. (2006). *Mindset: The new psychology of success.* Random House.

Edmondson, A. (2019). *The fearless organization: Creating psychological safety in the workplace for learning, innovation and growth.* John Wiley & Sons.

Ekman, P. (1997). Should we call it expression or communication? *Innovation in Social Science Research, 10*, 333–344.

Ekman, P. (2004). *Emotions revealed: Recognizing faces and feelings to improve communication and emotional life* (2nd ed.). Henry Holt.

Ekman, P., Camps, J., Davidson, R., & de Waal, F. (Eds.). (2003). Emotions inside out: 130 years after Darwin's The Expression of the Emotions in Man and Animals. *Annals of the New York Academy of Sciences, Volume 1000.* New York Academy of Sciences.

Eppich, W., Rethans, J. J., Teunissen, P. W., & Dornan T. (2016). Learning to work together through talk: Continuing professional development in medicine. In S. Billett, D. Dymock, & S. Choy (Eds.), *Supporting learning across working life. Professional and practice-based learning* (Vol. 16). Springer. https://doi-org.libproxy.temple.edu/10.1007/978-3-319-29019-5_3

Evans, A., McKenna, C., & Oliver, M. (2002). Self-assessment in medical practice. *Journal of the Royal Society of Medicine, 95*(10), 511–513.

Frederickson, B. (2003). The value of positive emotions. *American Scientist, 91*, 330–335.

Frederickson, B. (2009). *Positivity.* Crown.

Goldsmith, M., & Reiter, M. (2007). *What got you here won't get you there: How successful people become even more successful.* Hyperion.

Goleman, D. (2003). *Destructive emotions: A scientific dialogue with the Dalai Lama.* Bantam Books.

Goleman, D., Boyatzis, R., & McKee, A. (2002). *Primal leadership: Realizing the power of emotional intelligence.* Harvard Business School Press.

Goodwin, N. (2017). How important is information and communication technology in enabling interprofessional collaboration. *Journal of Health Services Research & Policy, 22*(4), 202–203.

Gordin, P. C., & Trey, B. (2011). Finding the leader within: Thoughts on leadership in nursing. *Journal of Perinatal & Neonatal Nursing, 25*(2), 115–118.

Gottman, J., Levenson, R., & Woodin, E. (2001). Facial expression during marital conflict. *Journal of Family Communication, 1*(2001), 37–57.

Hall, L., & Bodenhammer, B. (2002). *Mind lines: Lines for changing minds.* NeuroSematic Publications.

Hamm, A., Schupp, H., & Weike, A. (2003). Motivational organization of emotions: Autonomic changes, cortical responses, and reflex modulation. In R. J. Davidson, K. R. Sherer, & H. H. Goldsmith (Eds.), *The handbook of affective sciences* (pp. 187–211). Oxford University Press.

Hatfield, E., Cacioppo, J. T., & Rapson, R. L. (1993). *Emotional contagion.* Cambridge University Press.

Hu, Y., Parker, S., Lipsitz, S., Arriaga, A., Peyre, S., Corso, K., Roth, E., Yule, S., & Greenberg, C. (2016). Surgeons' leadership styles and team behavior in the operating room. *Journal of the American College of Surgeons, 222*(1), 41–51. DOI: 10.1016/j.jamcollsurg.2015.09.013

International Nursing Association of Clinical and Simulation Learning Standards Committee. (2021). Healthcare simulation standards of best practice™ simulation design. *Clinical Simulation in Nursing*, (1), 14–21.https://doi.org/10.1016/j.ecns.2021.08.009

Interprofessional Education Collaborative Expert Panel. (2016). *Core competencies for interprofessional collaborative practice: Report of an expert panel.* Interprofessional Education Collaborative.

Klenke-Borgmann, L., DiGregorio, H., & Cantrell, M. A. (2022). Role clarity and interprofessional colleagues in psychological safety: A faculty reflection. *Simulation in Healthcare*. doi: 10.1097/SIH.0000000000000662. Epub ahead of print. PMID: 35439796

Kolb, D. (1974). On management and the learning process. In D. Kolb, I. Rubin, & J. McIntyre (Eds.), *Organizational psychology: A book of readings* (pp. 27–42). Prentice Hall.

Kolbe, M., Weiss M., Grote, G., Knauth, A., Dambach, M., Spahn, D., & Grand, B. (2013). TeamGAINS: A tool for structured debriefings for simulation-based team trainings, *BMJ Quality & Safety*, 22, 541–553.

Landro, L. (2012, January 3). When nurses catch compassion fatigue, patients suffer. *Wall Street Journal*.http://www.wsj.com/articles/SB10001424052 9702047202045771288882104188856

Langer, E., & Imber, L. (1979). When practice makes imperfect: The debilitating effects of overlearning. *Journal of Personality and Social Psychology*, 37, 2014–2025.

Ludema, J. (2001). From deficit discourse to vocabularies of hope: The power of appreciation. In D. Cooperrider, P. Sorensen, Jr., T. Yaeger, & D. Whitney (Eds.), *Appreciative inquiry: An emerging direction for organizational development*(pp. 443–466). Stipes Publishing.

McEwen, B. (1998). Protective and damaging effects of stress mediators. *New England Journal of Medicine, 338*, 171–179.

McMurtry, A. (2007). Reinterpreting interdisciplinary health teams from a complexity science perspective. *University of Alberta Health Sciences Journal, 4*(1), 33–42.

National Academies of Sciences, Engineering and Medicine. (2019). *Taking action against clinician burnout: A systems approach to professional well being*. National Academies Press. http://doi.org/10.17226/25521

Nundy, S. (2021). *Care after COVID: What the pandemic revealed is broken in healthcare and how to reinvent it.* McGraw Hill.

Owen, H. (2008). *Open space technology: A user's guide.* Berrett-Koehler Publishers.

Peterson, L. (2009, August). *Healthcare and open space technology. The First Canadian Healthcare Conference*, Toronto. http://thefirstcanadianhealthcareconference .ca/index.php?/Healthcare-and-Open-Space-Technology

Salik, I., & Paige, J. T. (2021). *Debriefing the interprofessional team in medical simulation*. StatPearls Publishing.

Sampath, B., Rakover, J., Baldoza, K., Mate, K., Lenoci-Edwards, J., & Barker, P. (2021). *Whole system quality: A Unified approach to building responsive, resilient health care systems* (IHI White Paper). Institute for Healthcare Improvement. www.ihi.orgief.com

Sapolsky, R. (2004). *Why zebras don't get ulcers* (3rd ed.). Harper Collins.

Schot, E., Tummers, L., & Noordegraaf, M. (2020). Working on working together. A systematic review on how healthcare professionals contribute to interprofessional collaboration. *Journal of Interprofessional Care, 34*(3), 332–342, doi: 10.1080/13561820.2019.1636007

Senge, P. (2006). *The fifth discipline: The art and practice of the learning organization*. Doubleday.

Sharma, S., Boet, S., Kitto, S., & Reeves, S. (2011). Interprofessional simulated learning: The need for "sociological fidelity." *Journal of Interprofessional Care, 25*(2), 81–83. https://doi.org/10.3109/13561820.201 1.556514

Stone, D., & Heen, S. (2015). *Thanks for the feedback: The science and art of receiving feedback well*. Penguin Books.

Strazdins, L. (2000). Emotional work and emotional contagion. In N. Ashkanasy, W. Zerbe, & C. Hartel (Eds.), *Emotions in the workplace: Research, theory and practice* (pp. 232–250). Quorum Books.

Tannenbaum, S. I., Traylor, A. M., Thomas, E. J., & Salas E. (2021). Managing teamwork in the face of pandemic: Evidence-based tips. *BMJ Quality & Safety*, 30, 59–63.

Trzeciak, S., & Mazzarelli, A. (2019). *Compassionomics: The revolutionary scientific evidence that caring makes a difference*. Studer Group.

Wang, O. (2022, Sept. 29). *Physician burnout has reached distressing level, new research finds*. New York Times.

Wheatley, M. (2005). *Finding our way: Leadership for an uncertain time*. Berrett-Koehler Publishers.

Wheelan, S. A., Burchill, C. N., & Tilin, F. (2003). The link between teamwork and patients' outcomes in intensive care units. *American Journal of Critical Care*, 12, 527–534.

Whitney, D., Trosten-Bloom, A., & Radu, K. (2010). *Appreciative leadership: Focus on what works to drive winning performance*. McGraw Hill.

World Café. (2015). *A quick reference guide for hosting World Café*. www.theworldcafe.com

Xirasagar, S., Samuels, M. E., & Stoskopf, C. H. (2005). Physician leadership styles and effectiveness: An empirical study. *Medical Care Research and Review, 62*(6), 720–740.

© oxygen/Moment/Getty Images

Profiles in Collaboration

LEARNING OBJECTIVES

1. Analyze collaborative leadership behaviors in real-life situations.
2. Examine the meaning of collaborative cultures.
3. Employ positive communication and inclusive interprofessional dialogue to facilitate team function.
4. Identify boundary-spanning activities that support collaborative cultures.
5. Understand the dynamics of successful interprofessional healthcare teams.
6. Apply the concepts of collaborative leadership and positive communication to create a collaborative culture.

Every organization has its own unique spoken and unspoken rules that define the culture. Culture is often simply described as "the way we work around here." Cultures are formed and change through a variety of environmental events, leadership, and experiences. Dramatic and sometimes traumatic events impact the way cultures operate much the same way that the environment impacts personality in individuals. The way leaders respond to these events also shapes the culture. Edgar Schein (1986) defined culture using the following three levels:

1. **Artifacts:** These are the things you can easily see on the surface. How people behave is an artifact of culture.
2. **Espoused values:** These are the stated goals, philosophies, and values of an organization or group. Vision, mission, and values statements published on web pages, on posters, or in team charters are examples of espoused values.
3. **Basic assumptions and values:** These are the unconscious workings that underlie the core behaviors of a group. Shifting from a primarily hierarchical, disciplinary-centered culture to a more relationship- and patient-centered, collaborative culture is one of the primary challenges for healthcare systems.

Team cultures that value and actively seek each member's contribution can only inspire collaboration, commitment, and active engagement in the achievement of common goals (Wheatley, 2005, 2006; Whitney et al., 2010; Edmondson, 2019). Successful team leadership is, at its heart, an affirmation of the need for human beings to contribute and collaborate in a positive manner. Affirmative cultures are created and sustained through positive, rather than negative, dialogues, and groups that demonstrate a higher ratio of positive language tend to be more open to new ideas, more creative, and more productive. As feelings of self-efficacy emerge and grow, so does the perceived range of choices and possibility for action (Frederickson, 2003, 2009; Trzeciak & Mazzarelli, 2019).

REFLECTION: Cultural Cues

- What are some of the artifacts of your organization/team?
- What are the espoused values of your organization/team?
- If a friend was joining your organization/team and he wanted to know how to succeed, what would you tell him about the unspoken values and assumptions of your organization/team?

Like a pebble dropped into a pond, acts of affirmative leadership begin with the self and radiate out to impact other individuals, groups, organizations, and local and global communities. The result is the distribution of leadership behaviors beyond the designated leader and a facilitation of a culture of possibilities—a collective willingness to try new things and a more equal sharing of responsibility for goals and outcomes. Not surprisingly, this concept is associated not only with best practices in interprofessional healthcare teams but also in a wide range of highly profitable business endeavors (Anchor, 2012; Briskin et al., 2009; Edmondson, 2019; Fox, 2012; Institute of Medicine, 2001; Institute of Medicine, Gebbie et al, 2003a; Institute of Medicine, Greiner et al., 2003b; Pew Health Professions Commission, 1998; Spreitzer & Porath, 2012; World Health Organization, 2006; Zolno, 2007).

Creating and maintaining a collaborative culture is an important aspect of a professional orientation—no matter what the discipline or position in the organization. Members of high-performing teams perceive their work environment as having high levels of flexibility,

responsibility, standards, rewards, clarity, and team commitment. They feel that new ideas are welcomed, their expertise is trusted, accountability and excellence are the norm, expectations are clear, and there is a commonality of purpose (Spreier et al., 2006). The designated leader of the team sets the tone by modeling collaborative behaviors but also actively coaches team members by learning to listen, learning to ask powerful questions, and creating a safe environment based on trust and confidentiality (McKee et al., 2009; Edmondson, 2019).

Leaders facilitate the team's capacity to adapt by encouraging diverse perspectives. Members who take a leadership stance do so by practicing a professional assertiveness that allows them to offer their unique professional perspective while maintaining an active curiosity and actively soliciting the same from other team members. Opportunities for frequent, productive dialogue among team members facilitate the development of a common sense of purpose, which enables them to strategically leverage their unique professional and personal contributions. Interprofessional dialogue, at its most productive, is the art of thinking together and embracing different points of view (Isaacs, 1999).

Wheatley (2005) offers some provocative questions that can guide dialogue and help a healthcare team to define a unique, interprofessional culture that is strengthened by the diversity of its disciplinary parts:

- Who are we?
- What matters?
- What do people talk about and where do they spend their energy?
- What topics generate the most energy—positive or negative?
- What issues do people talk about most?
- What stories do they tell over and over?
- Is it possible to develop a sense of shared purpose without denying our diversity?
- Are there ways that we develop a shared sense of what is significant without forcing people to accept someone else's viewpoint?

The interprofessional healthcare team is, at its best, a community of practice—a community of practice that is sustained by ongoing and productive dialogue and continuous learning. Wenger (2006) describes a community of practice as "a group of people who share a concern or passion for something they do and learn how to do it better as they interact regularly" (p. 1). A community of practice has three distinguishing features: shared interest, engagement in information-sharing activities, and a development of shared resources such as experience, stories, and strategies for problem-solving that facilitate the learning of all participants—a shared practice. The conceptualization of the interprofessional healthcare team as a community of practice brings into high relief the basic values of patient- and relationship-centered practice that defines a collaborative interdisciplinary culture. Wenger (2006) notes a variety of activities that can help to span disciplinary boundaries and facilitate the development of a community of practice and a culture of collaboration. The examples in **Table 9.1** show how these activities can be used to support a collaborative interprofessional culture.

Cultures are often studied by listening to the collective stories told by the members of the organization. It is the tone of the day-to-day interactions that gives us insight into the web of values and behaviors that make up a culture. The following stories provide real-world perspectives about how people experience the cultures of their workplaces. Although each of their stories is unique, common themes include trust, open communication, empowerment, and patient-centered care.

A Technology-Enhanced Community of Practice[†]

Interprofessional education (IPE) focuses on collaborative practice, whereby students who learn together are able to create a

Table 9.1 Examples of Boundary-Spanning Activities That Support a Collaborative Culture

Problem-Solving: Can we get together to design a tool to evaluate the effectiveness of our caregiver training program?

Requests for Information: Where can I find the appropriate reimbursement codes for this diagnosis?

Seeking Experience: Has anyone dealt with a person who is a bilateral amputee with dementia?

Reusing Assets: I have a protocol that I have used with caregivers of persons with dementia. I can help you adapt it for use on your unit.

Coordination and Synergy: Can we collaborate on our patient education process and save time and resources?

Documentation Projects: What are some examples of best practices? What went right? How can we make that the norm?

Visits: Can we sit in on your in-service program? We think we may have similar needs.

Mapping Knowledge and Identifying Gaps: What information are we lacking for patients with left ventricular assist devices? We provide excellent cardiac rehabilitation, but this is a new patient group for us. What other individuals/groups should we connect with?

Data from Wenger, E. (2006). *Communities of practice: A brief introduction.* http://www.ewenger.com/theory

† Kathryn M. Shaffer, EdD, RN, MSN, CNE, CCFP, FNAP Associate Professor, Jefferson University, Philadelphia, PA.

knowledge-rich environment that shares the characteristics of a community of practice—common interest, community, and practice (Wenger, 1998). While students and educators see the value of IPE in clinical learning environments, many are challenged with competing schedules and course demands. Technology affords students learning environments that are easy to use, real-time, and collaborative, despite any logistical and scheduling barriers that may develop along the way. Technology can be used to develop the structured environments needed for students to develop the knowledge, skills, and attitudes of collaborative practice (Ho et al., 2010).

We conducted an action research study at one urban health science school to explore ways technology could be used to enhance IPE in a clinical service, allowing more students to collaborate and develop collaborative competency. The study was designed to use tools such as Google Docs and Google Hangouts for collaboration during clinical rounding on a patient care unit. Previous attempts to engage students and clinical faculty from a number of disciplines were not sustainable because of time and geographical constraints. Technology provided opportunities for students and faculty from multiple disciplines to transcend limitations imposed by logistics. With the use of Google Docs, nursing, pharmacy, medicine, and physical therapy students were able to join together to collaborate on a patient plan of care, which was later presented at bedside to the patient and surgeon. Members of the team collaborated on Google Docs throughout the day to add input or seek clarification of information. Students not physically at bedside were able to join the group through Google Hangouts.

Students stated that the experience was invaluable, and the faculty noted that the information exchange and collaboration of the students allowed for higher-order thinking and clinical reasoning. When asked about meaningful knowledge exchange, students felt that the technology enhanced their collaboration and how they functioned on a healthcare team.

An important subtheme from knowledge exchange was the awareness of patient safety during team exchanges.

- "I think the aspirin dose that my guy was on was real high . . . I brought it up to the team when they rounded and they didn't know why he was on such a high dose. So that question was definitely meaningful."
  —Nursing student

Students liked the collaborative tool Google Docs because it provided a platform for collaboration among team members in real time despite physical barriers.

- "With a Google Docs you could be anywhere and still get the information relayed."—Pharmacy student
- "It was kind of everyone coming together and doing everything at the same time . . . with the Google Docs you share it all with multiple people and we were all able to see it and provide input to it."—Physical therapy student

In this case, technology provided a communication tool that allowed students to see themselves as important members of an interprofessional community of practice.

The 12-Lead EKG†

An interprofessional team is one that incorporates all of the disciplines and professions

---

† Mary C. Sinnott, PT, DPT, MEd, FAPTA, Professor Emerita of Instruction, Program of Physical Therapy, Department of Health and Rehabilitation Sciences, College of Public Health Temple University, Philadelphia, PA.

required to move toward a patient's goals. An interprofessional team is like a 12-lead electrocardiogram (EKG). Much like a 12-lead EKG gives you 12 views of the heart, you get many different views of a case.

When I reflect on successful interprofessional teams that I have been a part of, the relationships and the time that we spent building relationships was key. It happened first of all with an understanding and consensus of what the patient had to accomplish. As a physical therapist, I do not have goals. There are no physical therapy (PT) goals; the patient has goals. I ask myself these questions: "What can I as a PT contribute to the patient's goals?" "How are others on the team looking at the goals?" In this ongoing conversation, you learn the perspectives of the other team members, and roles become clear. As a team you can answer the ongoing question, "Who on the team can best address the issues that are important to this patient?" Each team is unique to the setting or to an individual patient's needs. It is not enough to say, "I know what occupational therapy (OT) is." The question is, "What is the role of OT in this particular patient's care?" The more I know about how you practice as a profession, the better teammates we can be.

Formal team meetings contributed to the success of the team. But they were only one part of the success. The most productive interactions occurred when I was cotreating with someone, or I would ask for advice. You can leverage the expertise of your colleagues and generate creative solutions to problems.

As a leader, you really don't achieve anything on your own. You need to take care of relationships so you can take care of business. As both a team member as well as a leader, developing and maintaining relationships is day-to-day work that ultimately makes you successful.

I received a physical therapy consult for a 68-year-old woman who was admitted to the hospital from home. The chart said that she was independent at home but had recently experienced a change in her mental status. It was the end of the day, and the physicians were planning for her discharge that day. One might question the need for a physical therapy consult for a patient with mental status changes, but in this facility, a PT consult was standard procedure prior to discharge. The referral indicated that the patient was medically stable. I went to the patient's room and met the patient, her family, and the resident and medical student who were managing the case. Her daughter was crying. In a conversation away from the patient, the daughter said emphatically, "Mom cannot go home!" The daughter reported that her mother could not go home because she had started to fall as a result of her rapidly deteriorating mental status. The daughter could not continue to care for her mother. She had two small children, was working full time, and was recently divorced. She would come home and find her mom on the floor! As I assessed the patient, I demonstrated and explained to the resident and medical student. Her balance was horrific! She was clearly not safe! The decision was made that she could not go home. She was a clear fall risk. I admit that I also made an assumption about the patient's level of function based on the referral information. I went to the room thinking that PT would not be indicated and found that this patient clearly needed an aggressive PT program. I was able to convey that to the physician. Working together (and in consultation with the attending physician), the resident, the daughter, and I were able to stop an unsafe discharge. In this case, an intelligent conversation between disciplines led to a positive patient outcome. As I reflect on this case, I feel that it was successful because I introduced myself to the resident, was clear about what I had to offer as a physical therapist, and engaged the physician and the family (most importantly, the daughter) into an interprofessional conversation that focused on the needs of the patient.

Just-in-Time Communication†

On a well-functioning interprofessional team, the boundaries of the disciplines dissolve, and everyone works together for the benefit of the patient. Effective teams require the flow of communication among and between the disciplines. It is about creating a total picture of the patient. It requires that all team members be patient centered and holistic.

I feel that one key to the development and functioning of interprofessional teams lies in empowerment by the leadership. The leadership empowers the team by giving them the tools, training, and an understanding of what patient-centered care looks like. Leadership then models effective teamwork on a day-by-day basis in multiple circumstances.

A key blockage to effective interprofessional communication is day-to-day busyness. It creeps in. When staff are up to their eyeballs with discipline-specific tasks that they must attend to, communication becomes the most vulnerable to being compromised. For example, if a patient is exhibiting medical complications and the nurses are monitoring vital functions and medication levels and only communicating with the attending physician, then the opportunity to communicate what is happening with that patient to the rest of the team may be lost. The disciplines can then easily retreat into their silos. It is precisely at these crucial times when the patient's care is the most complicated that interprofessional communication is key.

Communication and teamwork techniques need ongoing training. Without well-planned training, the team does not work well, and the tendency is for professionals to revert back into previously learned modes of communication that are less effective and may compromise team functioning. If, for example, the physical therapist only reports on the patient's transfer status but doesn't mention that the patient told him during the session that her spouse just lost his job necessitating a social work consult, the progress of the whole team being able to address the identified need can be delayed and treatment and care can be adversely affected. If team members are encouraged to speak up, it becomes the team standard and the culture of the team. New members absorb this culture informally (by seeing it modeled) and formally (by attending training sessions), and it becomes self-perpetuating.

When new employees are brought aboard, they are oriented to our standards and expectations of teamwork and communication through an eight-hour workshop. If staffing allows for all new staff to be together, we break it up into sets of sessions that each focus on specific communication techniques and teamwork principles. Staff members participate in active sessions where they learn specific communication strategies involving various other disciplines, to see everyday issues from other perspectives. It gets staff up to speed with what we expect. It also empowers them to advocate for their patients and to speak up to other healthcare providers. We incorporate examples from our own unit to demonstrate the benefits of good teamwork and communication as well as the problems that can occur when communication and teamwork are lacking. We also reinforce that their input is highly valued.

We have developed an interprofessional communication system here that grew out of our teamwork and communication classes called Report Doc. All professionals for the shift-to-shift handoff use it. We now know everything about the patients from the perspectives of multiple disciplines, such as how they did in therapy, if there was a change in their diets (because they passed their swallow

---

† Sue Carol Verrillo, RN, MSN, CRRN, Nurse Manager, Department of Surgery, The Johns Hopkins Hospital, Baltimore, MD.

study), or perhaps a change in the amount of pain medicine that they require. For example, if the psychologist has determined that a particular patient does best if he is presented with only two choices per task, they would note this and team members could incorporate this strategy into their treatment sessions. Or if PT notes that the patient's ability to transfer has improved and she now requires only minimal assistance, nursing uses this information to assign staff for the next shift. This reporting system also has a column for anticipated needs and factors to watch for. Each team member is able to see the to-do list of his or her colleagues and again, communication is enhanced.

Creating a Research Community of Practice†

In the development of my research projects, I started reaching out to people in engineering to help me understand complex databases. I reached out to mathematicians to help me understand computational models. I brought in a biomechanic who had a better understanding of mechanics of motion. I brought my skills as a neuroscientist and my clinical point of view to the project. By assembling a team, we were able to ask more complicated questions and focus on researching a question that would have broad, practical implications.

A collaborative culture is also facilitated by organized social events, such as speed dating for researchers, that are designed to get researchers talking in a more informal way. During speed dating, pairs of participants speak for four minutes and are then moved on to the next table. These activities give participants an opportunity to know each other in a more relaxed environment and learn about the variety of research interests and networking possibilities in their community of practice.

Recently, I was part of an exciting interprofessional project. I secured a grant to support undergraduate students' research. I had six students from different majors ranging from computer science to kinesiology to psychology. I shared the grant with a faculty member from computer science. The research mentors in the project were also a diverse group—computer science, neuroscience, etc. We developed five projects that provided the students opportunities to utilize their special skills. For example, the computer science students developed the data collection programs that we needed. The psychology and kinesiology students collected data using the programs developed by the computer science students. I feel that much of the success of the project was due to the collaborative atmosphere that we created. Both my coinvestigator and I are very enthusiastic people and understood what we were trying to accomplish. He had the role of supporting the technology in the laboratory so that I could focus on the science. I know that I depended on his technological skills. We engaged in respectful sharing. We had weekly lab meetings where we shared both progress and engaged in group problem-solving as a team. At the conclusion of the grant, students were required to reflect on the experience. One student wrote, "Everybody should have this experience. It was the best experience of my education."

When I reflect on what makes a team successful, four factors come to mind: equanimity, open communication, common interests, and opportunities for personal development. The contribution of each

---

† Emily A. Keshner, PT EdD, Chief Research Officer, GraceFall, Inc., Emeritus Professor, Dept. of Health and Rehabilitation Sciences, Temple University Philadelphia, PA.

member on the team is respected. Many times, I was a member of a team that was made up of clearly senior and junior members. This did not mean that the senior members had the final say. The communication was characterized by intellectual sharing and openness. There was an ongoing process of learning. We were all learning at the same time and from each other.

How Do You Spell Successful Collaboration? R-E-S-P-E-C-T†

I value personal relationships. It is reflected in all of my team and group experiences. If you get to know people at a deeper level, it opens new channels of communication.

I strive to create a positive climate and empowering atmosphere. I love people, and I listen to my heart. I use an open communication style and give people permission to say what they want, and I listen. I hire managers who are also positive, respectful, good listeners, collaborative, and goal directed.

As a leader, I believe in getting people together. I look for commonalities, and I work diligently to create an atmosphere where collaboration and consensus are the norms. The following story is an example of how respect, collaboration, and consensus yielded successful outcomes.

I was a member of an interprofessional group that represented rehabilitation services in home care for the Joint Commission (formerly the Joint Commission on the Accreditation of Health Care Organizations, or JCAHO). The members of the group represented the American Occupational Therapy Association (AOTA), the American Physical Therapy Association (APTA), the American Speech and Hearing Association (ASHA), and three therapeutic recreation associations. There were 18 group members in total. I was the team leader and the only one who had a voice and a vote at the Joint Commission meeting. It was important that I went to the Joint Commission meeting with a clear idea of the ideas and feelings of each of the associations that I represented. We would meet as a group the night before the Joint Commission meeting to discuss the issues and achieve consensus. Before the meeting, I distributed an agenda. Each of the group members worked with their disciplinary associations and constituents to be sure that they accurately represented the issues. We would meet and work through the issues until we achieved 100 percent consensus and were able to speak with one voice. I feel that this process worked because each of the members of the group respected each other. We listened to each other—actively listened—and each member came to the meeting prepared. The day after the rehabilitation meeting, I joined nursing, medicine, and a number of other professions (there were 30 representatives in total) for a full-day Joint Commission meeting. I was the only voice for rehabilitation in home care at the table. As a team, we successfully lobbied for rehabilitation in home care. I feel that we were successful because each of the group members came prepared, respected each other, listened, and were committed to achieving consensus. We worked as a team. We understood that we were more powerful as a group than each of us would be individually. When I am a member or the leader of a successful team, I get excited! Building consensus by mobilizing a diversity of viewpoints can be both challenging and great fun! Setting a goal and seeing that goal met is thrilling.

---

† Rebecca Austill-Clausen, MS, OTR/L, FAOTA, Reiki Master, President of Complementary Health Works, Inc., Downingtown, PA.

Health Information Technology: A Tool for Collaboration†

A culture of collaboration is a fundamental element for the sustainable integration of health information technology (HIT) and health care. Making decisions about HIT should not be a top-down, isolated process but a collaborative process that takes into account the perspectives of information technology (IT) and clinical leadership, interprofessional healthcare team members, and patients. The digital infrastructure of a health system must be informed by the goals of the system and the needs of the stakeholders in that system. This is what is meant by the intentional design of HIT systems. If the overarching goal of the health system is to provide interprofessional, patient-, and family-focused care that is evidence based, the HIT tools must be designed to support those goals. Software and hardware has to support the usability of the electronic health record (EHR) system, interprofessional care planning, and evidence-based clinical documentation tools. For instance, evidence-based clinical practice guidelines; interprofessional care plans, evaluations, and assessments; and the patient's history must be designed so they support the individual needs of the professions, the integrated needs of the interprofessional team, and the unique needs of the patient and are accessible by all members of the team. Having workstations that are readily available on each unit for all professions to use enhances real-time documentation and improves team communication. This enables everyone to have immediate access to the information that is needed to care for the patient.

Since most members of the healthcare team provide and retrieve information at each juncture of the process of care, there are many opportunities to reinforce interprofessional collaboration when HIT is designed to support those processes. For instance, using a common tool for history taking can facilitate the sharing of patient information, improving collaboration, and reducing duplication. Developing an interprofessional plan of care is an opportunity for the integration of services and shared decision-making. Assessments and interventions can serve to clarify the unique contributions of each discipline, scopes of practice, role boundaries, and role overlap. Contextually relevant and intentionally designed HIT has the potential to become a "collective consciousness" for the interprofessional healthcare team, a vehicle that can support timely and consistent communication and collaboration among healthcare providers and healthcare consumers. The following is an example of this type of collaboration.

After transitioning from a paper charting system to an EHR, the healthcare team at University Hospital's Portage Medical Center in rural Ravenna, Ohio, made significant progress in advancing interprofessional collaborative care. The transition began with choosing an EHR with intentionally designed interprofessional documentation tools that supported the goals of the organization to achieve high-performance benchmarks and standards using evidence-based tools and to individualize the patient care experience based on patient preferences, life experiences, and customized patient goals.

Care is coordinated through a variety of health professionals, including nursing, respiratory therapy, physical therapy, occupational therapy, speech-language

---

† Tracy Christopherson, PhD, MS, BAS, RRT Co-Founder, MissingLogic; Lana F. Schuett, MSN, RN, ACNS-BC, Adult Clinical Nurse Specialist and Clinical Practice Model Site Coordinator, University Hospital Portage Medical Center, Ravenna, OH.

pathology, and nutritional services utilizing an interprofessional plan of care. The plan of care serves as a communication tool that enables the team to provide consistent, standardized, and individualized care. Evidence-based clinical practice guidelines form the foundation of the plan of care supporting the individual scopes of practice of each of the professions and the integrated and overlapping scopes of practice of the interprofessional team. This enables the team to utilize the appropriate resources at the right time. When scopes of practice overlap, the plan supports the team in providing consistent care while reducing duplication and repetition.

Utilizing the plan of care to advance interprofessional collaboration requires ongoing coaching and education. A variety of methods has been used, including focused education on care planning, rounding on the floors, and coaching. Staff have also been prepared to articulate how they use the plan of care to support evidence-based and individualized care when asked by regulatory bodies.

Care plan utilization and documentation compliance scores have increased 63 percent since the initial implementation, and an overall compliance rate of 96 percent has been maintained hospital-wide, which demonstrates how successful this initiative has been.

REFLECTION: Analyzing Team Cultures

- What levels of culture (artifacts, espoused values, and basic assumptions) are reflected in these stories?
- What characteristics of collaborative teams are in evidence?
- What characteristics of a community of practice are in evidence?
- What types of boundary-spanning activities are used?
- What leadership behaviors are used to foster a collaborative environment?
- Can you see these characteristics and behaviors at work in your setting? If not, how might they be employed?

REFLECTION: A Personal Profile in Collaboration

Think of a time when you chose to collaborate and the results were extremely positive.

- What was the situation?
- Why was it important for you to collaborate?
- What did you do to make the situation positive?
- What did others do to make the situation positive?
- What factors in the environment encouraged collaboration?
- What were the obstacles or challenges to collaboration?
- What practical advice would you give to someone to overcome obstacles or challenges to collaboration?
- How will this experience influence the way you approach other collaborative endeavors?

References

Anchor, S. (2012). Positive intelligence. *Harvard Business Review, 90*(1–2), 100–102.

Briskin, A., Erickson, S., Ott, J., & Callanan, T. (2009). *The power of collective wisdom and the trap of collective folly.* Berrett-Koehler.

Edmondson, A. (2019). *The fearless organization: creating psychological safety in the workplace for learning, innovation and growth.* John Wiley & Sons.

Fox, J. (2012). The economics of well-being. *Harvard Business Review, 90*(1–2), 79–83.

Frederickson, B. (2003). The value of positive emotions. *American Scientist, 91,* 330–335.

Frederickson, B. (2009). *Positivity.* Crown.

Ho, K., Jarvis-Selinger, S., Norman, C., Li, L., Olatunbosun, T., Cressman, C., & Nguyen, A. (2010). Electronic communities of practice: Guidelines from a project. *Journal of Continuing Education in the Health Professions, 30*(2), 139–143.

Institute of Medicine, Committee on Educating Public Health Professionals for the 21st Century; Gebbie, K., Rosenstock, L., & Hernandez, L. M. (Eds.). (2003a). *Who will keep the public healthy? Educating public health professionals for the 21st century.* National Academies Press.

Institute of Medicine, Committee on the Health Professions Education Summit; Greiner, A. C., & Knebel, E. (Eds.). (2003b). *Health professions education: A bridge to quality.* National Academies Press.

Institute of Medicine, Committee on Quality of Health Care in America. (2001). *Crossing the quality chasm: A new health system for the 21st century.* National Academies Press.

Isaacs, W. (1999). *Dialogue and the art of thinking together.* Doubleday.

May, N., Becker, D., Frankel, R., Haizlip, J., Harmon, R., Plews-Ogan, M., Schoring, J., Williams, A., & Whitney, D. (2011). *Appreciative inquiry in healthcare: Positive questions to bring out the best.* Crown Publishing.

McKee, A., Tilin, F., & Mason, D. (2009). Coaching from the inside: Building an internal group of emotionally intelligent coaches. *International Coaching Psychology Review, 4*(1), 35–46.

Pew Health Professions Commission. (1998). *Recreating health professional practice for a new century: The fourth report of the Pew Health Professions Commission.* Author.

Schein, E. H. (1986). *Organizational culture and leadership.* Jossey-Bass Publishing.

Spreier, S. W., Fontaine, M. H., & Malloy, R. L. (2006). Leadership run amok: The destructive potential of overachievers. *Harvard Business Review, 84*(6), 72–82.

Spreitzer, G., & Porath, C. (2012). Creating sustainable performance. *Harvard Business Review, 90*(1–2), 92–99.

Trzeciak, S., & Mazzarelli, A. (2019). *Compassionomics: The revolutionary scientific evidence that caring makes a difference.* Studer Group.

Wenger, E. (1998). *Identity in practice. Communities of practice: Learning, meaning and identity.* Cambridge University Press.

Wenger, E. (2006). *Communities of practice: A brief introduction.* http://www.ewenger.com/theory

Wheatley, M. (2005). *Finding our way: Leadership for an uncertain time.* Berrett-Koehler Publishers.

Wheatley, M. (2006). *Leadership and the new science: Discovering order in a chaotic world.* (3rd ed.). Berrett-Koehler Publishers.

Whitney, D., Trosten-Bloom, A., & Radu, K. (2010). *Appreciative leadership: Focus on what works to drive winning performance.* McGraw Hill.

World Health Organization. (2006). *The world health report 2006: Working together for health.* World Health Organization.

Zolno, S. (2007). Towards a healthy world: Meeting the challenges of the 21st century. *Linkage* (34), 14.

PART III

Building and Sustaining Collaborative Interprofessional Teams Activities

Activity 1: Mini 360-Degree Feedback Exercise

While self-reflection is an essential leadership behavior, you need to establish whether your view of yourself is consistent with those who you aspire to influence. A 360-degree perspective allows you to find out how you are viewed by your superiors, coworkers, and subordinates. Ask them the following questions regarding your effectiveness as a leader/member of a team. How do their answers compare to the answers you would give about yourself?

Similar answers will highlight areas of strength, while discrepancies will provide clues regarding areas for improvement.

- What should I do more of?
- What should I do less of?
- What could I do to contribute more positively to the team?

Activity 2: Social Identity

Social identity plays an important role in how we see ourselves and how we are seen by others. Social identity suggests that people have a natural inclination to identify with others they perceive are most like themselves. Becoming aware of how we see our own social identity is an important step in developing a more inclusive mindset.

Instructions

- Review the Social Identity List.
- Write down your answers to the three questions.
- Discuss highlights you feel comfortable sharing with one other person.
- Report out highlights of your conversation to the larger group.

Social Identity List

Age
Race
Ethnicity
National Origin
Language of Origin
Gender Identity/Expression
Sexual Orientation
Mental/ Physical Ability
Education Level
Socio-economic
Political Beliefs
Appearance
Religion
Personality Style
Workplace Experience
Professional Identity
Organizational Role
Other…

Answer These Questions

1. What social identity areas have shaped you?
2. Why might you experience some social identities more saliently than others?
3. What challenges, opportunities, and/ or privileges have your social identities brought to you?

Activity 3: The Art of Culture

Culture can seem like a difficult concept to grasp, yet we all know that each team (or organization) has a unique feel. This exercise helps you capture the feeling of your team (or organization) by drawing a picture of how you see it now and depicting your vision for a collaborative, interprofessional, and patient-centered culture for the future.

1. Think about how it feels to work where you work. Write some adjectives or short phrases that describe your culture or a metaphor that you have used that describes the culture.
2. Draw a picture of the current culture of your team or organization as it feels to you now.
3. Now think about how you would like the culture to be in the next three to five years. Write some adjectives or short phrases that describe your culture or a metaphor that you have used that describes the culture.
4. Draw a picture of the new culture.
5. Look at the two pictures. What do you think can be done to help change this culture? What is something you can change about your own behavior or attitude that may facilitate this change? How can you influence others to work toward positive culture change in your organization?

Activity 4: Checklist of Behaviors That Foster a Collaborative Culture

Check each item that applies to your team. The headings that have the most checks will indicate team strengths, while those with the fewest checks will indicate opportunities for improvement. How can you facilitate a collaborative interprofessional team culture?

Collaborative Culture Checklist

Role and Goal Clarification	
Encourages the process of goal, role, and task clarification	
Supports division of labor necessary to accomplish group goals	

Communicates in Order to Achieve Team Goals	
Encourages the adoption of an open communication structure where all member input and feedback is heard	
Promotes an appropriate ratio of the group task and members' emotional engagement and group process	
Promotes the use of affirmative dialogue	
Encourages use of effective conflict management strategies	
Employs effective problem-solving and decision-making procedures	

Develops Collaborative Team Norms	
Encourages the establishment of norms that support productivity, innovation, and freedom of expression	
Discourages any group tendency to over legislate individual behavior through the adoption of excessive or unnecessary rules	
Individuals voluntarily conform with norms that promote group effectiveness	
Welcomes diverse perspectives	

Takes Personal Responsibility for the Team's Success	
Members commit to personal and professional developments	
Members remain current in their respective fields	
Members actively draw on each other's expertise	
Members promote cohesion and cooperation	
Members take a positive approach to seeking solutions for the team's problems	
Members interact with others outside of the team in ways that promote the team's ability to interface within the larger organizational context	
Members have an understanding of group development and group process	

Employs Energizing Strategies	
Moves toward relationship building	
Engages team members on a personal level	
Makes time for reflection and personal renewal	
Stays appreciative and positive; discovers opportunities in challenges	

Index

Note: Page numbers followed by *f* or *t* represent figures or tables respectively